Study Guide to Accompany

Nutrition, Health, and Safety for Preschool Children

With Study Questions

Observation Activities

Application Activities

GLENCOE

McGraw-Hill

New York, New York
Columbus, Ohio
Mission Hills, California
Peoria, Illinois

Cover Photo Credits:

Background - Aaron Haupt Photography
Inset - Aaron Haupt Photography & Lane Avenue
        Horticultural Farm, The Ohio State University

Study Guide to accompany *Nutrition, Health, and Safety for Preschool Children*

Send all inquiries to
Glencoe/McGraw-Hill
936 Eastwind Drive
Westerville, OH 43081

ISBN 0-02-802092-8 Study Guide
ISBN 0-02-802089-8 Student's Edition

Printed in the United States of America

1 2 3 4 5 6 7 8 9 10   MAL   00 99 98 97 96 95 94

Co-developed by
Glencoe/McGraw-Hill
and Visual Education Corporation
Princeton, NJ

Contents

Introducing Nutrition, Health, and Safety

Match the descriptions on the left with the relevant terms on the right.
Write the letter of each correct answer in the space provided.

____ 1. The state of being poorly nourished for an extended
period of time

____ 2. Freedom from risk, harm, and injury

____ 3. The state of a person's overall physical, mental, and
emotional well-being

____ 4. The study and science of the foods people consume and
the physical processes involved in taking in and using
food

____ 5. The sum of the traits, characteristics, and defects that are
passed from parents to their children through genetic
mechanisms

____ 6. The condition that results when people do not eat
enough food containing essential nutrients

____ 7. The physical, economic, social, and cultural setting

____ 8. The condition that results when people consume too
much of one or more nutrients

____ 9. Substances in food that provide nourishment and help
the body function

a. environment

b. health

c. heredity

d. malnutrition

e. nutrients

f. nutrition

g. overnutrition

h. safety

i. undernutrition

Write answers to the following questions in the space provided.

10. List the three major factors that contribute to a child's well-being and
summarize their interrelationship.

_____

_____

_____

11. List the six major nutrients.

_____

_____

_____

12. Briefly describe the relationship between a person's age and his or her nutrient needs.

_____

_____

_____

_____

13. Why is sound nutrition so important in a young child's life?

_____

_____

_____

_____

14. Describe two factors that influence the food choices people make.

_____

_____

_____

_____

15. How can caregivers help ensure that children in their care are receiving adequate nutrition?

_____

_____

_____

_____

16. List three factors that affect a person's health.

_____

_____

_____

_____

17. List three traits that are inherited.

_____

_____

_____

_____

18. List the four types of settings that play a significant role in determining the level of a child's health.

_____

_____

_____

_____

19. What type of physical environment allows children to reach optimum levels of health and well-being?

_____

_____

_____

_____

20. How can caregivers protect and promote the health of children in their care?

_____

_____

_____

_____

21. What is the first responsibility of child care professionals?

_____

_____

_____

_____

22. What is the first step caregivers should take toward providing a safe environment?

_____

_____

_____

_____

23. List the most common hazards for young children.

_____

_____

_____

_____

24. What should caregivers do to reinforce safe behavior?

_____

_____

_____

_____

25. Explain what emergency preparedness involves in the child care setting.

_____

_____

_____

_____

26. Briefly summarize the interrelationship of nutrition, health, and safety as well as the effects of heredity and the environment.

_____

_____

_____

_____

Food Patterns for Healthy Development

Match the descriptions on the left with the relevant terms on the right.
Write the letter of each correct answer in the space provided.

_____ 1. The feeling of fullness or satisfaction that comes with eating

_____ 2. The beliefs, customs, knowledge, and habits that people share

_____ 3. The conditions around a child that include furniture, eating utensils, cleanliness, and all the child's encounters with food

_____ 4. A psychological desire to eat

_____ 5. A physical sensation that signals that it is time to eat

_____ 6. How, when, where, and how much food people eat

_____ 7. Foods common to a specific ethnic group

a. appetite

b. culture

c. ethnic foods

d. food environment

e. food patterns

f. hunger

g. satiety

Write answers to the following questions in the space provided.

8. Explain why it is important to promote a positive food environment.

_____

_____

_____

_____

9. How can you determine whether furniture and utensils are appropriate for a particular age group?

_____

_____

_____

_____

10. List three steps caregivers can take to promote cleanliness in the food environment.

_____

_____

_____

11. What is the difference between hunger and appetite?

_____

_____

_____

12. How often do most preschoolers need to eat?

_____

_____

_____

_____

13. Why should children eat a variety of foods?

_____

_____

_____

14. List at least four of the guidelines that caregivers should follow when preparing food for young children.

_____

_____

_____

_____

15. What can a caregiver do to respect the food preferences of a child?

_____

_____

_____

_____

16. How can caregivers use meals and snacks to encourage children to become more independent?

_____

_____

_____

_____

17. What is the best way to introduce children to new foods?

_____

_____

_____

_____

18. What factors help shape a child's food patterns?

_____

_____

_____

_____

19. How is the early food behavior of children related to their families?

_____

_____

_____

_____

Study Questions to Use with Chapter 2 ■ ■ ■   **7**

20. List some characteristics of modern families that may affect children's food behaviors.

_____

_____

_____

_____

21. What can caregivers do to help children deal with stress that affects their eating?

_____

_____

_____

_____

22. Summarize the main principles on which multicultural food education should be based.

_____

_____

_____

_____

23. How can a child care center incorporate multicultural food experiences in its program?

_____

_____

_____

_____

Name _____ Date _____ Class _____

Nutritional Needs of the Developing Preschooler

Match the descriptions on the left with the relevant terms on the right.
Write the letter of each correct answer in the space provided.

____ 1. A test performed to determine the amount of fat under the skin at specific locations on the body

____ 2. Propensities toward certain types of food preparation or certain groups of foods

____ 3. The tendency to use one hand over the other to perform fine motor tasks

____ 4. Tooth decay

____ 5. An instrument used to measure the amount of fat under the skin

a. caliper

b. dental caries

c. food preferences

d. hand preference

e. skinfold measurement

Write answers to the following questions in the space provided.

6. What should teachers do if a child's height or weight varies greatly from normal ranges for a significant period of time?

_____

_____

_____

7. Describe the principal changes in body proportions that a preschooler undergoes.

_____

_____

_____

8. Name three meal-related activities that preschoolers' newly developed motor skills allow them to perform.

_____

_____

_____

9. When children have mealtime accidents, such as dropping dishes or spilling food, how should teachers respond and why?

_____

_____

_____

_____

10. What newly acquired intellectual abilities allow preschoolers to learn about the basic food groups and to participate in cooking projects?

_____

_____

_____

11. According to the age-related method of determining energy needs, how many calories would a four-year-old need per day?

_____

_____

_____

12. What is the maximum recommended percentage of a preschooler's caloric needs that should be supplied by fats? Name three common sources of dietary fats.

_____

_____

_____

13. Which mineral is most often lacking from children's diets and why?

_____

_____

_____

_____

14. List three vegetables that are good sources of vitamin C.

_____

_____

_____

_____

15. Which types of meats should be limited in a preschooler's diet?

_____

_____

_____

16. What nutrients do enriched or fortified breads and cereals supply?

_____

_____

_____

17. What can teachers do to make food visually appealing to preschool children?

_____

_____

_____

18. What guidelines should a teacher follow when introducing a new food to a preschooler?

_____

_____

_____

19. Why is providing a choice of foods an important part of getting young children to eat?

_____

_____

_____

_____

20. What are two ways for teachers to limit preschoolers' intake of processed sugar?

_____

_____

_____

21. Why do the key principles of meal planning allow a child to have occasional meals and snacks that do not meet all nutritional guidelines?

_____

_____

_____

_____

22. How can teachers help counter the effects of television advertising on children's diets?

_____

_____

_____

_____

23. What can teachers do to encourage school-age children to eat the right kinds of snacks?

_____

_____

_____

_____

Name _____ Date _____ Class _____

Children with Special Nutritional Needs

Match the descriptions on the left with the relevant terms on the right.
Write the letter of each correct answer in the space provided.

_____ 1. An inherited disease that affects the mucus-producing glands of both the lungs and the digestive system

_____ 2. An inability to digest the sugar found in milk

_____ 3. The presence of excess lipids, including cholesterol, in the blood

_____ 4. A condition in which the body produces an inadequate amount of the hormone insulin

_____ 5. A condition in which a person does not have enough hemoglobin or red blood cells to carry oxygen from the lungs to all parts of the body

_____ 6. A condition in which the body's immune system reacts to a food substance as if it were an attacking organism

_____ 7. A condition in which a person is unable to metabolize phenylalanine properly

_____ 8. A condition that is characterized by skin inflammation and may be a symptom of a food allergy

_____ 9. The excessive storing of fat in the body

_____ 10. A condition in which the body lacks the enzyme(s) needed to make use of a particular food

a. anemia

b. cystic fibrosis

c. diabetes mellitus

d. eczema

e. food allergy

f. food intolerance

g. hyperlipidemia

h. lactose intolerance

i. obesity

j. phenylketonuria

Write answers to the following questions in the space provided.

11. List three possible causes of nutritional deficiencies.

_____

_____

_____

12. Why do children need more iron per pound of body weight than adults?

_____

_____

_____

13. What are two techniques for increasing the body's absorption of iron from food?

_____

_____

_____

14. Name three circumstances that may put children at risk of having a vitamin D deficiency.

_____

_____

_____

15. Name three pieces of evidence that support the conclusion that body weight is influenced by genetic factors.

_____

_____

_____

16. What have researchers found about the relationship between television viewing and obesity?

_____

_____

_____

17. What can teachers do to encourage obese children to participate in physical activities?

_____

_____

_____

18. Explain how hypertension is controlled in children with no other medical problems.

_____

_____

_____

_____

19. Why are allergic reactions to food most common during infancy? What is the best way to control a food allergy?

_____

_____

_____

_____

20. List four of the most common food allergens for young children.

_____

_____

_____

_____

21. What steps should caregivers take to ensure that a child is not exposed to a known food allergen at the child care center?

_____

_____

_____

_____

22. How should caregivers handle a food intolerance?

_____

_____

_____

_____

23. What are two difficulties that parents or caregivers may face when providing nutrition for a child with a developmental delay?

_____

_____

_____

_____

24. Why do low birth weight babies need more nutrients than heavier, full-term babies?

_____

_____

_____

_____

25. Explain why mothers of premature infants are encouraged to breast-feed.

_____

_____

_____

_____

Health Awareness and Special Needs

Match the descriptions on the left with the relevant terms on the right. Write the letter of each correct answer in the space provided.

_____ 1. Abnormal development of a fetus caused by the mother's use of alcohol during pregnancy

_____ 2. A condition caused by unusually strong discharges of electricity in the brain; commonly known as epilepsy

_____ 3. A process that stimulates the immune system to make substances that protect the body from specific infectious diseases

_____ 4. Persisting for a long time

_____ 5. A condition in which blood does not clot properly

_____ 6. A middle ear infection

_____ 7. A condition in which children suddenly and unexpectedly die in their cribs

_____ 8. Tests performed on apparently healthy people to detect disorders at an early stage

_____ 9. A condition in which swelling of lung tissues interferes with breathing

_____ 10. A condition in which red blood cells are misshapen and unable to carry enough oxygen to the body's tissues

a. asthma

b. chronic

c. fetal alcohol syndrome

d. hemophilia

e. immunization

f. otitis media

g. screenings

h. seizure disorder

i. sickle cell disease

j. sudden infant death syndrome

Write answers to the following questions in the space provided.

11. Explain why regular medical and dental checkups are important.

_____

_____

_____

12. Name three pieces of information that child care facilities typically keep on file about each child in their care.

_____

_____

_____

13. What is a medical release form?

_____

_____

_____

_____

14. What are the benefits of conducting a brief morning health check of each child in a child care facility?

_____

_____

_____

15. If a caregiver cannot reach a parent or emergency contact person when a child is sick, what should the caregiver do?

_____

_____

_____

_____

16. List the two emergency procedures in which all caregivers in a facility should be trained.

_____

_____

_____

_____

17. What are some common signs of a possible vision problem?

_____

_____

_____

18. What is strabismus? How can it be treated?

_____

_____

_____

_____

19. How can a child be affected if a hearing problem goes undetected?

_____

_____

_____

_____

20. List four chronic disorders that affect young children.

_____

_____

_____

_____

21. Describe what happens to a child during an asthma attack.

_____

_____

_____

_____

22. Why do children with hemophilia need to be protected from injury as much as possible?

_____

_____

_____

_____

23. What does the Americans with Disabilities Act of 1990 specify?

_____

_____

_____

_____

24. What health information do child care facilities typically require prospective employees to provide?

_____

_____

_____

_____

25. What is the correct technique for lifting a child or a heavy object?

_____

_____

_____

_____

Illness and Infectious Diseases

**Match the descriptions on the left with the relevant terms on the right.
Write the letter of each correct answer in the space provided.**

____ 1. A person or animal on which parasites live and from which they draw their nourishment

____ 2. A stage in all infectious illnesses in which a person starts showing nonspecific signs of illness

____ 3. An infection that can be passed from one person to another

____ 4. A person who may spread a disease to other people without ever showing symptoms of the disease

____ 5. Preventive measures people should take to avoid infection

____ 6. The stage of illness in which a person is definitely sick and shows symptoms typical of a specific infection

____ 7. Disease-causing organisms

____ 8. The stage of illness in which a pathogen multiplies inside the body without giving any signs that the person is infected

____ 9. A condition caused by organisms capable of entering the body and damaging tissue

____ 10. An illness for which certain occurrences must, by law, be reported to local or state public health agencies

a. acute stage

b. carrier

c. communicable disease

d. host

e. incubation period

f. infectious disease

g. pathogens

h. prodromal stage

i. reportable disease

j. universal precautions

Write answers to the following questions in the space provided.

11. List three reasons why children in child care settings are more at risk from infectious diseases than children who are at home.

_____

_____

_____

_____

12. What are viruses?

_____

_____

_____

_____

13. Explain briefly how immunization works.

_____

_____

_____

_____

14. Identify two factors that help determine whether a person exposed to an infectious disease will become ill.

_____

_____

_____

_____

15. List the four general ways in which communicable infections are transmitted.

_____

_____

_____

_____

16. What two practices in a child care center can help prevent the spread of infections transmitted by respiratory droplets?

_____

_____

_____

_____

Name _____ Date _____ Class _____

17. What is Hib disease and why is it dangerous?

_____

_____

_____

18. Explain how caregivers can prevent the spread of fecal-oral infections.

_____

_____

_____

19. What is giardia? Where does it originate and how is it spread?

_____

_____

_____

20. Describe the symptoms of conjunctivitis. What is the recommended treatment for the bacterial form of the disease?

_____

_____

_____

21. What can caregivers do to help control the spread of head lice?

_____

_____

_____

22. How is HIV spread? Name three common avenues of interpersonal contact that do *not* put a person at risk of becoming infected with the virus, and explain why they do not.

_____

_____

_____

_____

23. List four of the nine major childhood diseases for which vaccines are available.

_____

_____

_____

24. Give four examples of ways that caregivers can set up the physical environment of a child care center to minimize the spread of disease.

_____

_____

_____

25. What information should be included in a center's written policy on caring for sick children?

_____

_____

_____

Safe Environments

**Match the descriptions on the left with the relevant terms on the right.
Write the letter of each correct answer in the space provided.**

_____ 1. A situation in which a child climbs into an appliance, shuts the door, and is unable to open it from inside

_____ 2. Accidents that could have been foreseen and possibly prevented

_____ 3. Something that entices people to a restricted area or private property and may also pose a danger

_____ 4. An unintentional injury in which oxygen cannot get to the lungs because an object is covering the mouth and nose or there is pressure on the throat or chest

_____ 5. An area that is free of furniture and equipment and available for play

_____ 6. Suffocation by submersion in water or other liquids

_____ 7. A term used to describe a fabric or other material that is difficult to set on fire

_____ 8. Harmful or poisonous

a. attractive nuisance

b. drowning

c. entrapment

d. flame-retardant

e. mechanical suffocation

f. toxic

g. unintentional injuries

h. usable space

Write answers to the following questions in the space provided.

9. What has been the major cause of the dramatic decline in the death rate among children during this century?

_____

_____

_____

10. What is the single largest cause of injuries during childhood? What accounts for many of these injuries?

_____

_____

_____

11. Explain why infants are especially vulnerable to suffocation.

_____

_____

_____

12. What safety risk requires that babies be held when they are being fed?

_____

_____

_____

13. Between what ages are young children most likely to die from unintentional injuries? List two reasons why many accidents occur in this age group.

_____

_____

_____

14. Under what circumstances are accidents most likely to occur in a child care center?

_____

_____

_____

15. When should a car seat be placed facing the rear of a vehicle? When should it be placed facing the front?

_____

_____

_____

16. In what age group do most pedestrian fatalities occur? What accounts for this?

_____

_____

_____

_____

17. What is the principal difference between the method of preventing unintentional injuries in infants and toddlers and the method of preventing them in preschoolers and school-age children?

_____

_____

_____

18. Why do some school-age children knowingly participate in unsafe behavior?

_____

_____

_____

19. List the two causes of most bicycle accidents.

_____

_____

_____

_____

20. Identify three safety devices commonly installed in child care centers.

_____

_____

_____

_____

21. What qualities should caregivers look for when selecting toys for a child care center?

_____

_____

_____

_____

22. What types of art supplies should be avoided?

_____

_____

_____

_____

23. Describe how toddler and preschool playgrounds should be set up.

_____

_____

_____

_____

24. What are the pros and cons of choosing pea gravel, sand, or wood chips over rubber matting as a playground surface?

_____

_____

_____

_____

Safe Behavior and Emergency Response

**Match the descriptions on the left with the relevant terms on the right.
Write the letter of each correct answer in the space provided.**

_____ 1. A condition in which exposure to high temperatures for long periods of time causes dehydration and/or the loss of salts from the body

_____ 2. A nonaccidental injury or pattern of injuries to a child for which there is no "reasonable" explanation

_____ 3. The failure of a parent to provide for the physical care, safety, education, and emotional well-being of a child

_____ 4. A condition, often associated with injury, in which insufficient blood reaches important parts of the body

_____ 5. Verbally threatening, rejecting, ignoring, belittling, isolating, or placing unreasonable demands on a child

_____ 6. Inflammation of the skin, ranging from mild reddening to extensive blistering, caused by exposure to the sun

_____ 7. Sexual activity among members of a family who are not married to each other

_____ 8. The freezing of body tissues from exposure to cold temperatures

_____ 9. A form of abuse in which a child is exploited for the sexual gratification of an adult

_____ 10. Injuring a child by shaking, hitting, beating, burning, or performing other violent acts

a. child abuse

b. child neglect

c. emotional abuse

d. frostbite

e. heat exhaustion

f. incest

g. physical abuse

h. sexual abuse

i. shock

j. sunburn

Write answers to the following questions in the space provided.

11. List three general guidelines to follow to prevent injuries in a child care setting.

_____

_____

_____

_____

12. Why must safety rules for young children be more specific than those for older children?

_____

_____

_____

_____

13. What safety procedures should caregivers follow when children are involved in an activity that requires the use of appliances, tools, or other equipment not specifically designed for a child care classroom?

_____

_____

_____

_____

14. If a child's aggressive behavior goes beyond the normal level of preschool confrontation, what should the teacher do?

_____

_____

_____

_____

15. List three rules for safe playground play that caregivers should consistently enforce.

_____

_____

_____

_____

16. Explain why children are more susceptible than adults to dehydration.

_____

_____

_____

_____

17. What is a travel rope? How is it used?

_____

_____

_____

_____

18. List three safety procedures that child care centers can implement to help prevent the abduction of a child from the center.

_____

_____

_____

_____

19. What basic concepts can preschoolers be taught with regard to stranger safety?

_____

_____

_____

_____

20. Whose phone numbers should caregivers have on file for each child in their care?

_____

_____

_____

_____

21. What information do most injury or medical emergency reports include?

_____

_____

_____

_____

22. Describe basic first aid for a child who has burned her hand.

_____

_____

_____

_____

23. Describe basic first aid for a child whose foot is bleeding badly.

_____

_____

_____

_____

24. Explain why a case of child neglect is often easier to identify than a case of child abuse.

_____

_____

_____

_____

25. If you suspect child abuse and plan to report it, what information should you have handy?

_____

_____

_____

_____

26. List the three important concepts to teach children regarding child abuse.

_____

_____

_____

_____

Curriculum Design and Lesson Planning

**Match the descriptions on the left with the relevant terms on the right.
Write the letter of each correct answer in the space provided.**

_____ 1. Periods when one activity is ending and another is about to begin

_____ 2. A person's feelings, beliefs, or opinions about a person, object, or event

_____ 3. An expression of the intended outcome of a lesson

_____ 4. An approach to curriculum in which the teacher determines and leads the lesson or activity

_____ 5. The process of identifying goals and making plans to provide educational experiences

_____ 6. An approach to curriculum in which children are given opportunities to choose their own activities and decide for themselves how to explore new materials and pursue new experiences

a. attitudes

b. child-initiated

c. curriculum

d. instructional objective

e. teacher-directed

f. transition times

Write answers to the following questions in the space provided.

7. What are the two goals of nutrition, health, and safety education for young children?

_____

_____

_____

_____

8. What are the four basic elements of a preschool curriculum?

_____

_____

_____

_____

9. What can teachers do to help a child develop a positive self-concept?

_____

_____

_____

_____

10. Identify the five different types of skills a preschool curriculum can help children develop.

_____

_____

_____

_____

11. What attitudes toward people and experiences should an effective preschool curriculum try to encourage?

_____

_____

_____

_____

12. What can teachers do to promote positive social attitudes among children?

_____

_____

_____

_____

13. Name four of the five basic guidelines for planning an effective curriculum.

_____

_____

_____

_____

14. Give an example of a learning experience that uses a child-initiated approach.

_____

_____

_____

_____

15. How can teachers best structure a curriculum to help children learn?

_____

_____

_____

16. How should teachers respond to children who withdraw from active participation in activities?

_____

_____

_____

_____

17. List the five steps involved in preparing a lesson plan.

_____

_____

_____

_____

18. Name three basic nutrition, health, and safety concepts that can be taught to preschoolers.

_____

_____

_____

_____

19. What are three criteria that caregivers should use when evaluating potential topics to illustrate a concept?

_____

_____

_____

_____

20. Name two qualities of an effective instructional objective.

_____

_____

_____

_____

21. What are three reasons for evaluating a lesson plan?

_____

_____

_____

_____

22. When should lesson plans be reviewed and why?

_____

_____

_____

_____

23. In addition to the basic guidelines for planning an effective curriculum, name three other factors that should be considered when preparing lessons.

_____

_____

_____

_____

Approaches to Parent Involvement

**Match the descriptions on the left with the relevant terms on the right.
Write the letter of each correct answer in the space provided.**

_____ 1. A type of preschool in which parent governing boards make policy decisions and hire staff members

_____ 2. The exchange of messages between people

_____ 3. A restatement of another person's feelings or concerns made to show that the feelings are understood and valued

_____ 4. Watching and listening to classroom activities, usually without direct participation

_____ 5. Abilities to concentrate on what is being said and to participate actively in the communication process

a. communication

b. cooperative

c. listening skills

d. observation

e. reflective statement

Write answers to the following questions in the space provided.

6. List four factors that influence a child's ideas about nutrition before preschool.

_____

_____

_____

7. Name three methods of gathering information about children who are entering a child care program.

_____

_____

_____

8. What types of information should be freely exchanged between parents and teachers?

_____

_____

_____

9. Give an example of a parent-teacher exchange in which the teacher uses a reflective statement.

_____

_____

_____

_____

10. Explain why caregivers should be available to parents at drop-off and pickup times.

_____

_____

_____

_____

11. How should caregivers exchange private information with parents?

_____

_____

_____

_____

12. Why is it important for a center to make a copy of any written communication with parents?

_____

_____

_____

_____

13. Give three examples of the type of information that might be included on an infant's daily report form.

_____

_____

_____

_____

14. What type of information should teachers emphasize at parent-teacher conferences? Give an example.

_____

_____

_____

_____

15. What are three methods of sharing public information with parents?

_____

_____

_____

_____

16. What types of public information might child care centers put in fliers?

_____

_____

_____

_____

17. Why is it useful to put the daily menu on a separate sheet in a child care center's newsletter?

_____

_____

_____

_____

18. Give an example of a program that a preschool might sponsor for parents.

_____

_____

_____

_____

19. Explain why home visits are an effective way for caregivers to communicate with children and their parents.

_____

_____

_____

_____

20. What do parent contributions to newsletters, bulletin boards, and special events have in common?

_____

_____

_____

_____

21. What is the best thing that caregivers can do to gain parents' trust?

_____

_____

_____

_____

22. Identify the general ways in which parents can participate in the classroom.

_____

_____

_____

_____

23. Why is it important for caregivers to recognize privately and publicly the contributions of parent volunteers?

_____

_____

_____

_____

Name _____ Date _____ Class _____

Nutrition, Health, and Safety in Child Care

OBJECTIVES
- Identify ways that nutrition, health, and safety are interrelated.
- Identify practices that keep children healthy and safe in preschool.

SITUATION
Visit a child care center or family day care. Observe the physical setup of the room and the playground and practices that affect the health and safety of the children.

Type of child care setting _____

Age range of children observed _____

ASSIGNMENT

1. Observe snack time. Are tables washed before the snack is served? Are the children's hands washed? Do caregivers wash their hands?

_____

_____

_____

2. Observe the toys and other play materials in the room. Are they in good condition? Are the toys and play areas clean? If there is a water table, does the water look clean? Do any toys have broken parts or small pieces that a child might swallow?

_____

_____

_____

_____

3. Observe the children during indoor play. Do any children mouth a toy that has been in someone else's mouth? Do caregivers intervene to prevent this from happening? Do any children sneeze or cough near toys? Do children who are coughing seem less energetic or more irritable than other children?

_____

_____

_____

4. Observe the outdoor play area. What equipment is available? Describe the condition of the equipment. Do you observe any unsafe conditions?

_____

_____

_____

INTERVIEW

Interview a caregiver about the interrelatedness of nutrition, health, and safety. Note responses to the following questions.

5. In what ways do you find that nutrition, health, and safety concerns are interrelated?

_____

_____

_____

6. Under what conditions do you allow a child with a cold or cough to attend class?

_____

_____

_____

_____

Name _____ Date _____ Class _____

The Food Environment of a Child Care Setting

OBJECTIVES

- Describe how meals are prepared, served, and cleaned up in a preschool establishment.
- Describe the setting where the children eat their meals.

SITUATION

Visit a child care center or family day care and observe a meal being prepared and served.

Type of child care setting _____

Age range of children observed _____

ASSIGNMENT

1. Observe the preparations for a meal and describe what you observe. Is the meal prepared at the center or do children bring food from home? If prepared at the center, describe the kitchen facilities. Is there a separate staff in charge of meal preparation, or do the caregivers handle food responsibilities? Do food preparers wash their hands before handling food? Do they wear rubber gloves and/or hairnets? Where are the children when the meal is being prepared? If the children bring food from home, is it kept refrigerated?

_____

_____

_____

_____

_____

_____

_____

_____

2. Describe where the children eat their meal. Do they eat in the room where they have other activities or in a separate room or cafeteria? Is the eating area located away from toilet and diapering areas? Describe the furniture, dishes, and eating utensils used. Do the children eat at small tables with sturdy child-sized chairs? Are the dishes, glasses, and utensils made of disposable paper or plastic, or are they reusable? If they are reusable, how are they washed?

_____

_____

_____

_____

3. Describe other activities connected with the meal. Are tables wiped clean before the meal is served? If so, by whom? Do children help set the table? Do children and caregivers wash their hands before mealtime?

_____

_____

_____

_____

4. Describe how the meal is served. Do children line up and choose food from a variety of choices? Is food set out on tables with all children served identical meals? Do children pick up their lunch boxes from their cubbies and serve themselves? Do children sit in assigned seats, or can they choose their places? How many children sit at each table? Do caregivers sit with them? Is dessert served separately or with the meal? How are drinks served?

_____

_____

_____

_____

5. Describe cleanup. What role do children play in cleaning up after the meal? Does a special cafeteria staff clear the tables? What is the role of the caregivers in cleanup? What happens to leftover food?

_____

_____

_____

_____

INTERVIEW

Interview a caregiver about the center's mealtime routines. Note responses to the following questions.

6. If meals are prepared at the center, who chooses the menus? If meals are brought from home, are there any rules or guidelines on what should and should not be included? For instance, are children allowed to bring in cans of soft drinks?

_____

_____

_____

_____

_____

7. What is your own approach to encouraging children to try unfamiliar foods?

_____

_____

_____

_____

_____

8. During mealtime, do you try to set an example of healthful eating habits for the children? If so, in what ways? If not, what do you consider your role to be during mealtime?

_____

_____

_____

_____

_____

9. Find out whether meals other than lunch are served in the child care setting you observed. If so, what other meal or meals are served? Are additional meals offered as part of the regular program of the center, or are they part of extended care? How many of the children eat more than one meal a day at the center?

_____

_____

_____

_____

10. Find out what accommodations are made for children who do not eat certain foods because of their families' religious practices or for other reasons.

_____

_____

_____

_____

OBSERVATION
ACTIVITY
TO USE WITH
CHAPTER 3

The Nutritive Content of a Preschool Lunch

OBJECTIVES
- Identify the nutritive content of food served at a preschool lunch.
- Describe meal preparation at a preschool.

SITUATION   Visit a preschool where lunch is prepared on the premises. If possible, do not observe at the setting where you observed for Chapter 2.

Age range of children observed _____

ASSIGNMENT

1. Observe the meal being prepared. Describe how food is cooked. Is the meat baked, broiled, stir-fried, or prepared some other way? Are vegetables steamed or boiled? Are fruits served raw or cooked? For each dish, is it prepared from fresh, frozen, or canned ingredients? Do any of the menu items—for example, bread or drinks—arrive prepackaged or ready to eat?

_____

_____

_____

_____

2. List all the food and drinks that are served. Do not forget to include the extras, such as butter or margarine, condiments, and salad dressing.

_____

_____

_____

_____

3. Identify sources of carbohydrates, saturated and unsaturated fats, proteins, vitamins, minerals, and water in the meal.

_____

_____

_____

_____

_____

_____

4. Describe any alternative food items the children can select for their meal. Are there several choices for the main course and for drinks? If only one main course is served, are alternatives available for children who do not like or cannot eat the one choice?

_____

_____

_____

_____

_____

5. Identify what the children actually eat and drink. Do most children finish everything on their plates, or is a lot of food thrown away? What foods tend to be left over? Do more children finish the main course, bread, vegetables, fruit, or drink?

_____

_____

_____

_____

_____

Name _____ Date _____ Class _____

INTERVIEW

Interview the cook for the preschool. Note responses to the following questions.

6. Do you plan the menus, or are they given to you? If you plan them, please describe that process. If they are given to you, who plans them? Are you permitted to make changes in the menus provided?

_____

_____

_____

_____

_____

7. What nutrition guidelines do you follow when you prepare food? For instance, do you limit the amount of saturated fat you use in cooking?

_____

_____

_____

_____

_____

8. Do you try to introduce the children to foods from a variety of ethnic groups, or do you serve primarily those dishes you know the children are familiar with and enjoy? Please explain why you favor one approach over the other.

_____

_____

_____

_____

_____

9. Survey the children and caregivers at the center. Find out which are the favorite meals served at the center and which meals are least liked. Do the children and caregivers have similar likes and dislikes? Are favorite dishes healthful choices that are good sources of nutrients?

_____

_____

_____

_____

_____

_____

10. Describe the similarities and differences in the ways meals are prepared in this preschool setting and the one you observed for Chapter 2.

_____

_____

_____

_____

_____

_____

Name _____ Date _____ Class _____

Healthful and Safe Food in a Child Care Setting

OBJECTIVES
- Identify ways that food served in a child care setting contributes to the health of the children.
- Describe the safety procedures followed in food preparation and cleanup in a child care setting.

SITUATION

Visit a child care center or family day care and observe lunch being prepared and eaten. If children bring in their own lunches, observe snack time instead.

Type of preschool setting _____

Age range of children observed _____

ASSIGNMENT

1. Observe the meal or snack being prepared. Identify sources of fat. What foods are fried? What foods are cooked or served with butter or margarine? Is fat and/or skin removed from meat or poultry? Are processed meats served? Is low-fat or regular mayonnaise used to prepare salads? Are regular or low-fat frozen desserts served? Food labels will help identify sources of fat.

_____

_____

_____

2. Note which foods and drinks contain added sugar. Is chocolate milk served? If canned fruit is used, is it packaged in fruit juice or syrup? Does the cook use sugar in preparing any food? Check food labels to see whether yogurt, applesauce, peanut butter, salad dressing, spaghetti sauce, or other packaged foods contain added sugar.

_____

_____

_____

3. What food groups are represented in the meal or snack? Does most of the food fall in the Bread, Cereal, Rice, and Pasta Group? Are there foods from all five food groups? How many items fall in the Fats, Oils, and Sweets category? (Peanut butter made with added sugar falls in the Meat Group; a peanut butter cookie may have some nutritive value but would be counted among the Sweets.)

_____

_____

_____

_____

_____

4. Identify all fruits and vegetables that are available to the children as part of the meal or snack. Is there a good source of vitamin C? Is there a good source of vitamin A? Is there a good source of complex carbohydrates?

_____

_____

_____

_____

_____

_____

5. Observe the food handlers who prepare the lunch or snack. Note the following:

Food Safety Precautions	Yes	No
Wash hands before starting to work with food		
Wear rubber gloves and hairnets		
Thaw frozen foods in refrigerator or microwave oven		
Wash all fruits and vegetables		
Wash tasting spoons before using again		
Wash knives and other utensils between uses with different foods		

6. Describe the cleanup procedures. Are cutting boards, knives, other utensils, and pots and pans thoroughly cleaned? How is perishable food handled? What is done with leftover food?

_____

_____

_____

_____

_____

_____

INTERVIEW

Interview a food handler or caregiver about health and safety issues related to food. Note responses to the following questions.

7. Are there any food groups that you find children tend to dislike? How do you encourage them to eat foods from this group?

_____

_____

_____

_____

_____

8. In planning meals and/or snacks, do you find the Food Guide Pyramid or USDA planning guides to be of help? If so, in what ways? If not, why not? What other nutrition resources or dietary guidelines do you use?

_____

_____

_____

_____

_____

_____

FOLLOW-UP ACTIVITIES

9. Find out what is served for lunch or a snack at this child care setting over a five-day period. Use the Food Guide Pyramid to assess what food groups are represented and in what quantities. Over the course of the week, do the children receive a well-balanced, varied, and moderate diet?

_____

_____

_____

_____

_____

10. Telephone several child care centers that serve meals. Ask them to send you sample menus. Evaluate the meals for fats and added sugars. Is there an excess of fried foods or luncheon meats? Are there many sweetened baked goods or fruits in syrup?

_____

_____

_____

_____

_____

Name _____   Date _____   Class _____

Language Development of Young Children

OBJECTIVES
- Describe the language development of infants, toddlers, and preschoolers.
- Describe ways that caregivers help promote language development.

SITUATION

Visit a child care setting that accepts infants, toddlers, and preschoolers. Observe the language development of the children and the verbal interactions of the caregivers with the children.

Type of child care setting _____

ASSIGNMENT

1. Observe a group of infants. Note their age range. Note what sounds they make. Do any of the infants say any recognizable words? If so, what are they? Do the infants appear to be trying to communicate? If so, what makes you think so? Are there indications that the infants understand more words than they can say? For example, do they respond to their own names?

_____

_____

_____

_____

2. Observe the caregivers interacting with the infants. Note their use of language. What do they say to the infants? Note their tone of voice and the complexity of the vocabulary and sentences they use. Do they speak to the infants the same way that they speak to adults? Do they use a different tone of voice than they use with adults?

_____

_____

_____

_____

3. Observe a group of toddlers. Note their age range. Observe the language skills of the toddlers. Are some toddlers easy to understand whereas others are still babbling? Do any toddlers speak in two- or three-word phrases? What food words do you hear them using?

_____

_____

_____

_____

4. Observe the caregivers interacting with the toddlers. Note what they say to the toddlers. Note their tone of voice and the complexity of the vocabulary and sentences they use. Do you observe them expanding what the toddlers say? What differences do you notice in the caregivers' use of language with the infants and with the toddlers?

_____

_____

_____

_____

5. Observe a group of preschoolers. Note their age range. Observe the language skills of the preschoolers. Do they speak in complete sentences? How well do they describe their needs and wants? Does language figure more prominently in their play activities than it does in the toddlers'?

_____

_____

_____

_____

6. Observe the caregivers interacting with the preschoolers. Note what they say to them. Note their tone of voice and the complexity of the vocabulary and sentences they use. What differences do you notice in the caregivers' use of language with the infants, the toddlers, and the preschoolers?

_____

_____

_____

_____

INTERVIEW

Interview the director of the center or one of the caregivers about the language development of the children and ways that caregivers promote language development. Note responses to the following questions.

7. What materials and activities do you use to enhance and encourage the language development of the children? What similarities and differences are there in your approach when you are working with infants, toddlers, and preschoolers?

_____

_____

_____

_____

8. Are there any children in the center who come from homes where a language other than English is spoken? Are there any differences in the development of their English? Do you speak with them differently than you speak with the native speakers of English?

_____

_____

_____

_____

9. Do you believe in using baby talk—simplified language—when you speak to very young children? Why or why not?

_____

_____

_____

_____

_____

Observation Activity to Use with Chapter 5 ■ ■ ■

FOLLOW-UP ACTIVITIES

10. Ask the parents of two or three preschoolers at what age their children began to speak and what the children's first words were. Record their answers.

_____

_____

_____

_____

_____

_____

11. Read an article in a professional journal about the language development of young children. Note the name of the journal, the title of the article, and the author, as well as the date of publication. Summarize the information in the article.

_____

_____

_____

_____

_____

_____

Name _____ Date _____ Class _____

Feeding Infants in a Child Care Setting

OBJECTIVES
- Describe how infants' nutritional needs are met in a child care setting.
- Describe safety and sanitation practices that protect the health of infants.

SITUATION
Visit a child care center or family day care where infants as young as six weeks of age are cared for. Observe the infants when they are fed by caregivers.

Type of child care setting _____

ASSIGNMENT

1. Observe preparations for feeding infants under three months of age. Does each infant have a bottle that parents send in, or are bottles provided by the center? Is formula sent in by parents or provided by the center? Are any infants fed expressed breast milk? Are bottles washed just before being filled? If bottles are warmed, how is this done? How does the caregiver check the temperature of the formula or breast milk before feeding it to an infant?

_____

_____

_____

2. Observe infants under three months old being fed. How many infants in this age group are in this setting? How many caregivers are available to feed them? Do caregivers follow a schedule or feed each infant on demand? How much time do caregivers spend with each infant? How many times during a feeding is each infant burped? When an infant is being fed, is the caregiver free to focus his or her attention exclusively on the infant? Identify what is fed to each infant. Do any mothers come in to breast-feed their infants?

_____

_____

_____

3. Observe older infants being fed. Identify the number and ages of the infants. Describe the setting. Are some infants fed in infant seats? Are some infants able to sit up in high chairs? How many children are fed at the same time? How many caregivers feed the infants?

_____

_____

_____

_____

_____

4. Describe the process of feeding the older infants. What do they eat? Is each child fed different food brought from home, or are the children all fed the same food? If baby food from jars is used, do caregivers feed children directly from the jar or scoop a small amount at a time onto a separate plate? Are any children given finger food to eat by themselves? Is any food heated?

_____

_____

_____

_____

_____

5. Observe cleanup. What is done with unused food and unfinished milk or formula? When and how are the infants' hands and faces washed? When and how are the high chairs and infant seats cleaned? When and how is the floor cleaned? What are the infants doing while caregivers are cleaning up?

_____

_____

_____

_____

_____

INTERVIEW

Interview a caregiver who feeds infants. Note responses to the following questions.

6. What difficulties are there in feeding infants? Do you find it a challenge to cope with the feeding schedules of several infants, or do you find that the infants generally conform to a manageable routine?

_____

_____

_____

_____

7. Do you keep track of how much and what each infant eats? Do parents often want this information? Do you have a policy on what foods to introduce in what order, or do parents tell you what to feed their children?

_____

_____

_____

_____

8. In your experience, what foods pose a choking or other food-related hazard? How do you limit these hazards? What do you do if a parent sends in food you feel poses a safety hazard?

_____

_____

_____

_____

_____

FOLLOW-UP ACTIVITIES

9. Ask two mothers of young infants whether they chose to breast-feed their infants. If not, why not? If so, how long did they breast-feed or how long do they plan to continue? Ask whether they ever express their milk. Find out whether placing their children in child care affected their decisions about whether to breast-feed and how long to breast-feed.

_____

_____

_____

_____

_____

10. Ask a parent of an older infant at what age the infant was introduced to solid foods. Ask what foods the parent first fed the child and how the infant responded to the introduction to solid foods.

_____

_____

_____

_____

_____

Name _____   Date _____   Class _____

Feeding Toddlers in a Child Care Setting

OBJECTIVES
- Describe the physical setting where toddlers are fed.
- Describe mealtime routines for toddlers in a child care setting.

SITUATION
Visit a child care setting and observe toddlers getting ready for and eating lunch.

Type of child care setting _____

ASSIGNMENT

1. Describe the physical setting in which lunch is served. Is there a cafeteria or separate room where meals are served, or are they served in the classroom? Do the toddlers eat with older and/or younger children? Do caregivers sit and eat their meals with the children? Describe the tables, chairs, dishes, and utensils the toddlers use.

_____

_____

_____

_____

2. Observe the class getting ready for the meal. Is there a particular activity—for example, a song, a story, or a poem—that signals it is time to eat? Where do children and caregivers wash their hands before the meal? Who sets the table? Who brings food to the table? Do children have difficulty settling down to eat?

_____

_____

_____

_____

3. Observe the toddlers eating their lunch. Are finger foods served? Do the children use utensils? How are drinks served? Describe the help the children receive from caregivers and how much they do on their own. Are younger toddlers fed by caregivers?

_____

_____

_____

_____

_____

4. Describe serving sizes. Do most of the children taste every food offered? How many children finish every food offered? Do any children ask for second helpings? How do caregivers respond if children ask for seconds of one food without having tried another?

_____

_____

_____

_____

_____

5. Listen to conversations that take place during the meal. Do caregivers talk to the children about the food? Do they encourage the children to try different foods? If caregivers eat with the children, do the caregivers eat some of every food offered? What else do caregivers talk to the children about during the meal? Do children talk to each other about the meal? If children bring lunches from home, do they ask to try food from each other's lunches?

_____

_____

_____

_____

_____

Name _____ Date _____ Class _____

6. Observe what happens after the meal. Are children expected to wait until everyone is finished eating before leaving the table? If children are allowed to leave the table when they finish, what do they do while other children are still eating? How long does the meal last? Who cleans up after the meal? Do children help?

_____

_____

_____

_____

_____

INTERVIEW

Interview a caregiver about mealtime concerns. Note responses to the following questions.

7. What strategies have you used successfully to encourage reluctant toddlers to eat a wider variety of food?

_____

_____

_____

_____

_____

8. Toddlers are becoming adept at eating independently but are also at risk of choking. What do you do to minimize the risk of choking? Do you know what to do if a child begins to choke? Have you ever had to deal with a situation in which a toddler was choking?

_____

_____

_____

_____

_____

9. Are there children in the class who have restrictions on what they can eat? If so, how have you accommodated their special needs?

_____

_____

_____

_____

_____

FOLLOW-UP ACTIVITIES

10. Cookbooks that focus on cooking for children and cooking columns in parents' magazines offer many suggestions for preparing healthful food that appeals to children. Select a recipe that is healthful and easy to prepare. Cite the source, copy the recipe, and explain why it is likely to appeal to toddlers.

_____

_____

_____

_____

_____

11. Survey the children's menu choices at three restaurants, including one fast-food restaurant. Evaluate the nutritive content of the meals. Do they include a variety of fruits and vegetables? How many foods from the Bread, Cereal, Rice, and Pasta Group are offered? Do fried foods and processed meats dominate the choices?

_____

_____

_____

_____

_____

_____

Name _____   Date _____   Class _____

Feeding Preschoolers in a Child Care Setting

OBJECTIVES
- Describe mealtime routines for preschoolers in a child care setting.
- Identify the nutritive content of a meal served to preschoolers.

SITUATION

Visit a child care center or family day care where lunch is provided and observe preschoolers preparing for and eating lunch.

Type of child care setting _____

ASSIGNMENT

1. Observe the children preparing for the meal and describe the procedure. How is the handwashing routine handled? Do preschoolers help prepare the food? Do they set the table? Do they bring food to the table or help serve the food?

_____

_____

_____

_____

2. Describe the lunch served to the children. How closely does the meal conform to the meal pattern for preschoolers shown in the chapter text? Is milk served with the meal? Does the meal include meat or a meat alternative, such as peanut butter, cheese, or cooked dry beans? How many fruits and vegetables are included? Is bread, rice, cereal, or pasta part of the meal?

_____

_____

_____

_____

3. How are serving sizes determined? Are children given premeasured servings of each food? Does a caregiver dish out the food, estimating the amounts? Is food served family style at the table, with children helping themselves?

_____

_____

_____

_____

4. Indicate whether each child is offered amounts that satisfy the meal pattern specifications for each category of food:

Food Category	Measure	Yes	No
Milk	¾ cup		
Meat or meat alternate			
Meat/poultry/fish OR	1½ ounces		
Cheese OR	1½ ounces		
Egg OR	1		
Cooked dry beans and peas OR	⅜ cup		
Peanut butter or other nut or			
seed butters OR	3 tablespoons		
Nuts and/or seeds	¾ ounce		
Vegetable and/or fruit (2 or more)	½ cup total		
Bread or bread alternate	½ slice		

5. How much do the children eat? Is there a particular food they all finish? Is there a particular food most of them leave unfinished? What do you think accounts for these patterns?

_____

_____

_____

_____

6. Observe the caregivers during the meal. Do they eat with the children? Do they eat a reasonable amount of each food? Do they seem to enjoy the food and enjoy eating with the children? What do caregivers and children talk about during the meal?

_____

_____

_____

_____

7. Observe what happens after the meal. What role do preschoolers play in the cleanup routine? What role do caregivers play? Describe the general mood of the class.

_____

_____

_____

_____

INTERVIEW

Interview a caregiver about feeding preschoolers. Note responses to the following questions.

8. Please describe two cooking or other food-related activities you have done with the children.

_____

_____

_____

_____

9. What nutrition information do you teach the children?

_____

_____

_____

_____

10. Please describe the role food plays in birthday and holiday celebrations at your child care facility. Do you permit food that you discourage at other times to be served on special occasions?

_____

_____

_____

_____

FOLLOW-UP ACTIVITIES

11. Think about the foods you liked and disliked when you were a child. Was there any food you hated? Was there any food you loved? Do you remember ever wanting to eat the same food over and over? Do you still like and dislike these same foods? In what ways have your food preferences changed over the years?

_____

_____

_____

_____

12. Teachers' and parent's magazines offer many suggestions for cooking activities to use with preschool children. Select an activity that involves preparing a healthful food. Cite the source and describe the activity. Explain what the activity will teach children about nutrition.

_____

_____

_____

_____

Name _____ Date _____ Class _____

Children with Special Nutritional Needs

OBJECTIVES

- Identify foods that may cause problems for children with special nutritional needs.
- Describe ways that caregivers accommodate the special nutritional needs of preschoolers.

SITUATION

Visit a child care center or family day care where meals are prepared and served to the children. Observe mealtime.

Type of child care setting _____

Age range of children observed _____

ASSIGNMENT

1. List what is served at the meal. If children are able to choose between several main courses, side dishes, and drinks, list all the choices.

_____

_____

_____

_____

2. Do any of the items served include substances such as eggs, wheat, corn, soybeans, chocolate, or peanuts that young children are often allergic to or have an intolerance for? List these foods. Is there a sufficient variety of choices so that children who have to avoid these substances can select suitable alternatives?

_____

_____

_____

_____

3. Are any foods served that may be inappropriate for children who are overweight? If so, identify the foods and explain why they are inappropriate. Suggest alternatives that can replace these foods.

_____

_____

_____

_____

_____

_____

4. Are any foods served that may cause problems for children with diabetes or other conditions? Identify these foods and the related problems.

_____

_____

_____

_____

_____

_____

5. Find out from caregivers whether any children are on restricted diets. Note what these children eat at this meal. Is food available to them on the regular menu, or are they served a separate meal?

_____

_____

_____

_____

_____

_____

INTERVIEW

Interview a caregiver about the special nutritional needs of children. Note responses to the following questions.

6. Give some examples from your work of children with special nutritional needs. What special accommodations do you make for these children?

   _____

   _____

   _____

   _____

   _____

7. What is your policy on foods that are high in sugar and fats and low in nutritive value? Do you allow these foods to be served on special occasions, such as birthdays and holiday celebrations? Do you allow them to be served as snacks?

   _____

   _____

   _____

   _____

   _____

FOLLOW-UP ACTIVITIES

8. Most of the food commercials that are aired during children's television programming promote products that are high in fats and sugar. One exception is the advertisement campaign for milk. Choose a healthy food product and create an advertisement for that product.

   _____

   _____

   _____

   _____

9. Look at the recipes in two issues of a parenting magazine. How many of the recipes are for desserts? How many are for main courses? Are the majority of the recipes high in nutritive value with a minimum of fats and added sugar? How many recipes include eggs, wheat, chocolate, or other common allergens among the ingredients? Identify the magazines you used.

_____

_____

_____

_____

_____

Name _____ Date _____ Class _____

The Health of Children and Caregivers

OBJECTIVES

- Describe the general health of the children and caregivers in a child care setting.
- Describe ways that information about health is communicated to parents, children, and caregivers.

SITUATION

Visit a child care center or family day care before and during pickup time and observe the overall health of the children and the caregivers and ways that information about health is communicated.

Type of child care setting _____

Age range of children observed _____

ASSIGNMENT

1. Observe the overall health of the children in the class. Do a majority of the children appear to be healthy? Note the number of children who are coughing, sneezing, or have runny noses. Note other signs of illness.

_____

_____

_____

_____

2. Observe the overall health of the caregivers. Are any caregivers coughing or sneezing? Do the caregivers appear to be in good health?

_____

_____

_____

_____

3. Observe the class for 20 minutes. Note any comments caregivers make regarding health practices. Do caregivers remind children to cover their mouths when they cough or to use tissues when they sneeze? Do caregivers discuss the importance of handwashing before eating?

_____

_____

_____

_____

4. Observe parents picking up children at the end of the day. Note any comments caregivers make concerning the health of the children. Note any questions parents ask caregivers about the health of their children.

_____

_____

_____

_____

INTERVIEW

Interview a caregiver about health-related issues. Note responses to the following questions.

5. Have you ever brought the need for vision, hearing, or other screening to the attention of a parent? What made you suspect there was a problem?

_____

_____

_____

6. What information about health is included in the curriculum?

_____

_____

_____

_____

Name _____ • _____ Date _____ Class _____

Limiting the Spread of Germs

OBJECTIVES
- Describe ways that the physical setup of a classroom can help limit the spread of germs in a child care setting.
- Describe other ways that caregivers can limit the spread of germs in a child care setting.

SITUATION
Visit a child care center or family day care and observe the physical setting and arrangements for toileting and feeding the children and for rest time.

Type of child care setting _____

Age range of children observed _____

ASSIGNMENT

1. Survey the room. If there is a diaper-changing area, is it located well away from the food preparation area? Is the room well ventilated? Where are the toileting and handwashing facilities for the children? Where are they for the caregivers?

_____

_____

_____

2. Observe children using the bathroom. Is there a time set aside for using the bathroom, or do children use the bathroom as needed? What assistance do caregivers give children? Do they make sure that the children wash their hands after using the bathroom? If caregivers assist the children with toileting, do they wash their own hands after helping each child?

_____

_____

_____

3. Survey the play area. Do the toys look clean? Do the play surfaces appear to be clean? Does the dress-up area contain hats?

_____

_____

_____

_____

4. Observe the children at play. Do you observe any instances where children put toys into their mouths or cough on toys that are then used by other children? Do you observe any other interactions that might promote the spread of germs? Do caregivers intervene in these instances?

_____

_____

_____

_____

5. Observe rest time, if there is one. Note the position of the children. Are they close enough to be breathing in each other's faces?

_____

_____

_____

_____

6. Do children have individual cubbies in which to store their coats and belongings? Are the children's belongings kept fairly separate by this means, or do coats and hats end up in a pile?

_____

_____

_____

_____

Name _____ Date _____ Class _____

INTERVIEW

Interview a caregiver about ways to limit the spread of illness. Note responses to the following questions.

7. Do you find that parents have a tendency to send children to school when they are obviously not well? What do you do when this happens?

_____

_____

_____

_____

_____

8. Explain what procedures you follow when a child becomes ill while at school.

_____

_____

_____

_____

_____

9. How often do you wash the toys and the play areas in the room?

_____

_____

_____

_____

_____

Observation Activity to Use with Chapter 11   ■ ■ ■

FOLLOW-UP ACTIVITIES

10. Find out whether the center where you observed has a handbook that lists the center's policies concerning illness. Summarize the policies. Does the center permit teachers or other staff members to administer medication sent from home? Does the center require proof of immunization before accepting a child for enrollment?

_____

_____

_____

_____

_____

_____

11. In some communities, there are child care services especially set up to care for mildly ill children. Find out whether this type of service is available in your area. Where is it located? How much does it cost? Who runs it?

_____

_____

_____

_____

_____

_____

_____

Creating a Safe Physical Environment

OBJECTIVES

- Identify ways to make the physical environment in a child care setting safe for children.
- Identify differences in safety concerns and equipment for children of different ages in a child care setting.

SITUATION

Visit a child care center or family day care and conduct a safety survey. Arrange to be there to observe drop-off or pickup time.

Type of child care setting _____

Age range of children observed _____

ASSIGNMENT

1. If this is a facility where children arrive by car, stand in the parking lot at drop-off or pickup time and note whether children are placed in car seats, booster seats, or seat belts. Are any children allowed to sit in the car without passenger restraints? If this is a facility where the children come by bus, observe the buses during drop-off or pickup time. Are the buses equipped with seat belts? Are all children buckled in?

_____

_____

_____

_____

_____

_____

2. If children walk to and from the facility, observe them arriving or leaving. Note the care with which the children are escorted across the street and in the vicinity of traffic. Are infants and toddlers carried or transported in strollers? Does an adult hold the hand of each older child? Are any of the children difficult to restrain from crossing the street when it is not safe to do so?

_____

_____

_____

_____

3. Conduct a safety survey of the room. Complete the checklist below.

Indoor Safety Survey	Yes	No
Electrical outlets covered with safety plugs		
Cleaning supplies, medications, and caregivers' belongings locked out of reach of children		
Shelves, cabinets, and heavy furniture anchored to walls		
Toys sturdy, with no small detachable parts or sharp edges		
All areas of room clearly visible		
All art supplies nontoxic (coded AP or CP)		
Smoke and carbon monoxide alarms, fire extinguishers, and emergency lighting in room		
Windows equipped with window guards and safety glass		
All stairways equipped with safety gates		
All houseplants nonpoisonous		

4. Observe children indoors at play or engaged in another activity for 10 to 15 minutes. Note what if anything they put in their mouths. Toys? Crayons? Paint? Clay? How do caregivers respond if children put toys and other materials in their mouths?

_____

_____

_____

_____

5. Conduct a safety survey of the outdoor facilities. Complete the checklist below.

Outdoor Safety Survey	Yes	No
Playground area fenced		
Ground covered with impact-absorbing material		
Swings with flexible rather than rigid seats		
Adequate space around large pieces of equipment		
All play areas visible		
Outdoor play areas located away from busy streets and other hazards		
Separate play spaces with appropriate equipment for different age groups		

6. Observe children outdoors at play for 10 to 15 minutes. If play areas for different age groups are not separated, do children try to use equipment that is inappropriate for their ages or abilities? How do caregivers respond if this happens? If older children ride tricycles or bicycles, do they wear helmets?

_____

_____

_____

_____

INTERVIEW

Interview a caregiver about the importance of safety considerations in a child care setting. Note responses to the following questions.

7. Explain how you provide an environment with materials and equipment that stimulate and challenge the older children while protecting the younger children from materials and equipment that would pose a hazard to them.

_____

_____

_____

_____

8. National performance standards developed jointly by the American Public Health Association and the American Academy of Pediatrics require at least 35 square feet of usable indoor space for each child in care. Have you had the experience of caring for children in a facility where there was insufficient space for the number of children? How did this affect the children? How did it affect your ability to care for the children?

_____

_____

_____

_____

_____

FOLLOW-UP ACTIVITIES

9. Find out what safety inspections, if any, are required for licensed child care facilities in your state. Is the child care center or family day care where you observed a licensed facility?

_____

_____

_____

_____

_____

10. Call four child care centers and ask what type of impact-absorbing material they each use under their playground equipment. Ask why this was the material chosen. Is one type of material more common than others? Why?

_____

_____

_____

_____

_____

Name _____ Date _____ Class _____

Safe Behavior Patterns

OBJECTIVES
- Describe ways that caregivers ensure the safety of children in a child care setting.
- Describe ways that caregivers enforce safety rules in a child care setting.

SITUATION

Visit a child care center or family day care and observe behaviors and arrangements that promote safety in the facility and safety rules enforced by caregivers.

Type of child care setting _____

Age range of children observed _____

ASSIGNMENT

1. Observe access to the facility. Do parents and visitors have to check in with anyone when they enter the building? Would an unauthorized visitor have easy access to this facility?

_____

_____

_____

_____

2. How many caregivers are responsible for the children you observe? How many children are in the class or family day care? Does this seem like an adequate amount of supervision? Why or why not? Is the ratio of caregivers to children within the guidelines recommended in your text?

_____

_____

_____

_____

3. Observe caregivers supervising the children. Describe any rules of behavior that you hear caregivers mention—for example, "Wait for John to get off the swing." Are the rules worded in positive terms? Are they easy to understand?

_____

_____

_____

_____

_____

4. Describe what happens when a conflict develops between two children. At what point does a caregiver intervene? Describe how the conflict between the children is resolved.

_____

_____

_____

_____

_____

5. Observe on the playground. Describe the weather conditions. Describe the way children are dressed. Are all children dressed appropriately for the weather? If it is hot and sunny, are the children wearing hats and sunscreen? If it is cold, are they wearing hats and gloves?

_____

_____

_____

_____

_____

Name _____ Date _____ Class _____

INTERVIEW

Interview a caregiver about the importance of safe behavior and emergency preparedness in a child care setting. Note responses to the following questions.

6. What training have you had in first aid or emergency response? If you have not had any such training, who on the staff is trained in emergency care? Have you ever had to deal with a medical emergency as a caregiver? Describe what happened to the child and what you did to deal with the immediate situation and to get proper medical attention for the child.

   _____

   _____

   _____

   _____

7. What emergency procedures do you have in case of a fire? Do you have regular fire drills with the children? If not, why not?

   _____

   _____

   _____

   _____

8. What precautions do you take to ensure that only authorized adults pick up children from your care? Have you ever refused to allow a child to leave with an adult who came for the child?

   _____

   _____

   _____

   _____

FOLLOW-UP ACTIVITIES

9. Survey two or three child care centers in your area. Ask administrators how they screen job applicants to make sure they do not hire people who have criminal records or who are likely to cause intentional harm to the children in their care. Summarize your findings.

_____

_____

_____

_____

_____

_____

10. Find a first-aid book. Read the section on recognizing the signs of concussion. Summarize the information. If you suspect that a child has a concussion, what steps should you follow?

_____

_____

_____

_____

_____

_____

Curriculum Planning

OBJECTIVES
- Identify ways that nutrition, health, and safety are incorporated into the preschool curriculum.
- Describe a nutrition, health, or safety lesson or activity.

SITUATION

Arrange to visit a preschool when the class will be involved in a nutrition, health, or safety lesson or activity. Plan to arrive before the lesson or activity begins.

Age range of children _____

ASSIGNMENT

1. What activity preceded the lesson or activity you are observing? Are the children given a transition time to change their focus from one activity to the next? Does it take the teacher a while to get the children settled down?

_____

_____

_____

_____

2. Where are the children situated during the lesson or activity? Do they begin as a group seated on the floor and then move to their seats to work on the activity? Do they move freely through an activity station?

_____

_____

_____

_____

3. What materials does the teacher use in the lesson or activity? What materials do the children use?

_____

_____

_____

_____

4. How much choice do the children have in determining the details of this lesson or activity? For instance, if the children are doing an art project, do they have a choice of colors? Media? Subjects? How much is predetermined by the teacher?

_____

_____

_____

_____

5. Describe the nutrition, health, or safety topic the teacher is focusing on and the teacher's method of presenting the topic. Does the teacher present a formal lesson or introduce the topic through related activities? Does the teacher make a variety of materials available to the children and let them explore the materials on their own?

_____

_____

_____

_____

6. Does the lesson or activity seem appropriate for the interest level and attention span of the children? Are they eager to participate? How long does the lesson or activity last? Do the children seem to understand the material? Do they need a lot of guidance to complete the activity successfully? Do they seem to enjoy the lesson or activity?

_____

_____

_____

_____

7. What physical skills are involved in completing this lesson or activity? What cognitive skills? What social skills?

_____

_____

_____

_____

INTERVIEW

Interview a caregiver about curriculum planning. Note responses to the following questions.

8. Were you pleased with the lesson or activity on nutrition, health, or safety? Why or why not? What changes would you make before doing this lesson or activity again?

_____

_____

_____

9. Will the topic covered in the lesson or activity observed today be covered again some other time? If so, in what way? Have you already introduced this topic to the children? If so, what other activities have you done with the children on this topic?

_____

_____

_____

10. Do you write formal lesson plans? If so, how far in advance do you make your plans? How closely do you follow them once they are made? If you do not write formal lesson plans, explain your approach to planning.

_____

_____

_____

FOLLOW-UP ACTIVITIES

11. Ask to see a copy of a teacher's lesson plans for a week. Summarize the topics covered. Do the plans include instructional objectives? If you were asked to be a substitute teacher in that class for a day, would you be able to work from these lesson plans? Why or why not?

_____

_____

_____

_____

_____

12. Read an article about curriculum planning in a professional journal such as _Young Children_ or _Child Development_. Summarize the main points of the article. Include the name of the journal, the author and title of the article, and publication date. If possible, find an article that discusses a curriculum approach to a nutrition, health, or safety topic.

_____

_____

_____

_____

_____

Name _____ Date _____ Class _____

Parent Involvement in the Child Care Setting

OBJECTIVES
- Identify ways that parents are involved in preschool classrooms.
- Identify ways that caregivers communicate with parents of preschool children.

SITUATION
Visit a child care center and observe parent involvement in a classroom. Make sure that a parent will be in the class on the day you observe.

ASSIGNMENT

1. Explain what the parent is doing in the class. Is the parent participating in a birthday celebration? Making a presentation related to his or her job or cultural background? Assisting with a special project?

   _____

   _____

   _____

2. Describe the interaction between the parent and the teacher. How often do the parent and teacher consult with each other? Is one of the adults following the lead of the other, or are they operating independently? Do the two adults work well together?

   _____

   _____

   _____

3. Describe the interaction between the parent and the children. Does the parent pay special attention to his or her own child? Does the parent try to give equal attention to all the children? How does the child react to having his or her parent in the room? Does the parent attract special attention from the other children?

   _____

   _____

   _____

4. Observe indications of parent involvement at the center. Is there a bulletin board with announcements and news items aimed at parents? If so, do most of the notices come from the center's staff or from parents themselves? Do parent volunteers work in the office?

_____

_____

_____

_____

INTERVIEW

Interview a caregiver about parent involvement in the class and about communicating with parents. Note responses to the following questions.

5. Explain your policy on parent participation in the classroom. Do parents work in your classroom on a regular basis? If not, do parents come in to share special knowledge or to participate in other ways? Do you find that children are distracted when parents are in the room?

_____

_____

_____

_____

6. Does the center send home a newsletter on a regular basis? Do you send home a separate newsletter as well? If so, how often? How else do you routinely communicate with parents?

_____

_____

_____

_____

Name _____ Date _____ Class _____

Nutrition, Health, and Safety Concepts

Read the passage below and answer the questions that follow.

It is the first week in September. For many children at the Westover Child Care Center, this is their first day of preschool. Eliza Green, teacher of the three-year-olds, meets the children and their families at the door, greeting familiar faces and saying a few words to each of the new children.

During morning circle time, Eliza tells the children that she would like to discuss what they can do about safety at school. She asks whether anyone knows what safety is.

The children respond eagerly: "It's so you don't get hurt." "It's so nobody throws something and gets a bump on his head." "It's not falling down."

Eliza goes on to explain ways of preventing accidents at school, including not climbing on the tables and chairs and not throwing things. She explains that picking up toys at cleanup time helps keep people from tripping over them. She also talks about being calm during fire drills.

Eliza then spends a few minutes talking about health procedures in class. She asks the children what they think they should do if they have to sneeze or cough at school, and they suggest: "Don't sneeze on somebody!" "Cover your face!" Eliza briefly explains the reasons for these precautions and shows the children where the tissues are kept. She also explains the routines for using the bathroom and for washing hands. She thanks the children for listening and moves on to some circle games.

At lunchtime, the children sit at the tables, sing a song, and begin to eat. While they are eating, Eliza explains that the children should stay in their seats until they are through eating because it is not safe to walk around the room with food in their mouths. She tells them that, although they do not have to finish everything in their lunch boxes, they should try everything. Finally, she asks them not to share food with the other children.

At the end of the day, Eliza makes notes about her discussions with the children. She also plans some other activities for dealing with nutrition, health, and safety topics in the weeks to come. In the meantime, she decides to observe how well the children's behavior at the center follows the guidelines she has provided.

1. What safety hazards is Eliza concerned about when she stresses picking up toys and not walking with food in one's mouth?

_____

_____

_____

2. Eliza is concerned about the children spreading illnesses by failing to wash their hands frequently enough. How can she reinforce this concept throughout the year so that the children learn it thoroughly?

_____

_____

_____

_____

3. Eliza does not insist that the children finish all the food in their lunch boxes, but she would like them to try each item. Do you agree with this policy? Why or why not?

_____

_____

_____

_____

4. Children often enjoy sharing things with friends. What problems might arise when children share food they have brought from home for lunch?

_____

_____

_____

_____

5. Do you think Eliza's discussions of nutrition, health, and safety issues were appropriate for a group of three-year-olds? Why or why not? List any changes or additions you would suggest.

_____

_____

_____

_____

Scheduling Meals and Snacks

Read the passage below and answer the questions that follow.

Donna is head teacher of the three-year-old class at the High Street Children's Center. The center opens at 7:30 A.M., and breakfast is available for the children who arrive early. All the children are served a snack about 10:00, lunch around noon, and another snack at 3:00 P.M. This schedule seems to suit most of the group, but there are two children who frequently complain of being hungry.

Jarrod usually arrives at the center at around 8:30 A.M. and immediately begins asking whether it is snack time yet. He has trouble settling down to play or listening to the teachers explain what the class is going to do. Jarrod says that he eats breakfast before he comes to school. Donna has noticed that Jarrod's behavior improves after the morning snack but that he doesn't eat much at lunchtime, when he seems to be in a hurry to leave the table and play.

Olivia also arrives around 8:30 and often complains that she is hungry. When asked whether she ate breakfast, Olivia usually replies that she wasn't hungry at breakfast time. However, after the 10:00 snack, Olivia becomes cheerful, and the rest of her day goes well.

Donna decides to talk to the parents of these two children. She wants to find out more about the children's morning routines at home and about their eating patterns, and she wants the parents to be aware of the situations.

Jarrod's mother tells Donna that Jarrod is constantly complaining about being hungry and asks for snacks all day long. She always gives him something. Every morning she serves him a bowl of cereal with milk, which he eats while she is getting dressed for work. He usually doesn't finish his cereal, and he doesn't eat much supper at night—just more of his "snacks."

Donna suggests that it might be a good idea to encourage Jarrod to eat fewer snacks and eat more at meals. To help him eat more at breakfast, she suggests adding some variety and mentions various breakfast foods that children seem to like. She also asks whether someone in Jarrod's family could eat breakfast with him to encourage him to eat a full meal and to set an example.

Olivia's father says that he offers his daughter breakfast every school morning but that she never wants anything. She does, however, eat breakfast on weekends about an hour after she wakes up. Donna suggests that it might help to wake Olivia a littler earlier on school mornings to give her time to develop an appetite before she leaves home. Alternatively, her father could bring her to the center a bit earlier so she could have breakfast with the early arrivals. Then she would be ready to begin the day.

1. Why do you think Donna considered these hunger patterns to be a problem?

_____

_____

_____

_____

2. Explain how the schedule for meals at home seems to differ for each of these two children from the schedule at school. How do these differences affect the children?

_____

_____

_____

_____

3. Donna suggested that Jarrod should learn to eat more substantial meals and fewer snacks. Do you think this is good advice for a child with Jarrod's pattern of frequent snacks? Why or why not?

_____

_____

_____

_____

4. Suggest some other questions about Olivia's eating patterns at home that Donna might ask to learn more about the situation.

_____

_____

_____

_____

5. Jarrod and Olivia both told their teachers when they felt hungry at school. What other signals in a child's behavior might indicate that the child needs to eat?

_____

_____

_____

_____

Name _____ Date _____ Class _____

The Use of Vitamin and Mineral Supplements

Vitamins and minerals are essential for children's good health and development. Children can get most of the vitamins and minerals they need by eating a variety of foods. Some people believe that their children will benefit from additional vitamin and mineral supplements. The following paragraphs outline two opposing views of the use of vitamin and mineral supplements. Read the passage and answer the questions that follow.

VIEW I. Proponents of the use of vitamin and mineral supplements contend that many children do not get all the vitamins and minerals they need from food. They point out that children who develop strong food dislikes (such as those who refuse milk or vegetables) and children who have food allergies may be lacking in some vitamins and minerals. These proponents also note that dietary restrictions followed for cultural or religious reasons may limit sources of certain nutrients. This is the case with some vegetarian diets. Even children who eat healthful diets most days, may have days when they do not eat well. Supplements, proponents say, provide a steady source of vitamins and minerals that may be missing from a child's diet.

Some proponents favor supplement use of only certain vitamins and minerals—for example, the water-soluble vitamins, which are not stored in the body. Other proponents favor supplement use under certain circumstances, such as during a growth spurt or during and following an illness.

VIEW II. Those opposed to the use of vitamin and mineral supplements include many health professionals who feel that such supplements are not necessary for children. They emphasize that a varied diet that includes recommended servings of food from the five food groups should provide all the nutrients a child needs. They also point out that nutrients found in food are often better absorbed by the body than the nutrients in supplements. They believe that the best long-term approach to improving children's vitamin and mineral intake is to help children develop good eating habits.

Opponents also note that supplements may contain dangerously high levels of certain vitamins and minerals. The fat-soluble vitamins, for example, are stored in the body and high doses from vitamin supplements can cause these vitamins to accumulate, possibly to levels that are harmful.

1. How do vitamin and mineral supplements differ nutritionally from foods that contain the same vitamins and minerals?

_____

_____

_____

2. Do you think it is important for caregivers to know which children in their care are given vitamin and mineral supplements at home? Why or why not?

_____

_____

_____

_____

3. Name some of the vitamins found in milk. What other foods containing these vitamins could a caregiver offer to a child who eats no dairy products?

_____

_____

_____

4. Give examples of two minerals that are important to children's growth and development. Do you think there might be cases in which a child would need supplements of these minerals? Explain your answer.

_____

_____

_____

5. In your opinion, what advice should a caregiver offer to parents who ask whether they should give vitamin and mineral supplements to their child?

_____

_____

_____

_____

Planning Meals for Preschoolers

Read the passage below and answer the questions that follow.

The Greenvale Nursery School is planning to offer lunches for the children who attend the full-day program. In the past, the school provided only snacks, and children had to bring lunch from home. To assist the new kitchen staff in planning menus, Eva Mercado, the director of the school, is preparing a list of foods that the children would enjoy.

Eva consults the Food Guide Pyramid so that her lunch menus will reflect current nutritional recommendations for daily servings of each food group. According to the pyramid, the greatest number of daily servings should come from the Bread, Cereal, Rice, and Pasta Group. For this reason, Eva's menus include at least one food from this group every day.

To gather ideas for foods that the children like, Eva meets with Karen Mullen's class of four-year-olds. Eva asks the children to name their favorite foods to get the discussion going. This produces a varied list of foods, including yogurt, cheese, peanut butter, bananas, pizza, tacos, ice cream, and hot dogs. She then asks the children what breads, cereals, and pastas they like and what their favorite rice dishes are. The children come up with a long list that includes bagels, pita bread, tortillas, cornflakes, spaghetti, macaroni, and rice pilaf.

Eva draws up sample lunch menus based on the Food Guide Pyramid and her discussion with the children. She bases each meal on one or more choices from the Bread, Cereal, Rice, and Pasta Group, along with servings of foods from the other food groups. Many of the dishes combine foods from one or more groups. Eva takes the children's preferences into account by proposing foods such as low-fat versions of pizza and tacos. She suggests a variety of fillings and breads for sandwiches and nutritious sauces for pastas. She also lists various ways of serving fresh fruits and vegetables.

When the lunch program based on these suggestions begins, Eva sends weekly menus home to the parents. Eva observes the children's reactions to the lunches and asks their families for comments on the menus. She and the kitchen staff coordinate the responses they receive with the food pyramid guidelines to make lunches nutritious and enjoyable for the children.

1. Is the Food Guide Pyramid a good resource to use in planning lunches? Why or why not?

_____

_____

_____

2. What beverage should Eva's school provide to the children at lunchtime? What are the nutritional benefits of that beverage?

_____

_____

_____

_____

3. Eva included a great deal of variety in her sample menus. Do you think this is a good idea? Would it be wiser to repeat a few of the children's favorite meals over and over? Why or why not?

_____

_____

_____

_____

4. Eva is providing information to parents about foods served to the children at lunchtime. Why is this important?

_____

_____

_____

_____

5. Suppose a child complains at lunchtime one day that she does not like any of the foods served. What do you think the teachers at this school should do?

_____

_____

_____

_____

Name _____ Date _____ Class _____

Development and Self-Feeding Skills

Read the passage below and answer the questions that follow.

Ryan is four years old and has been attending the Ocean View Child Care Center since he was three months old. During that time, Ryan has grown and changed in many ways. He is taller and heavier, and his body proportions have changed. He has acquired a variety of skills. As a result, what he eats and how he eats have evolved since he first came to the center.

When he was three months old, Ryan was held in a caregiver's lap and bottle-fed. At this early stage, he participated in his meals by sucking eagerly when he was hungry and turning his head away when he was full. When he was about five months old, Ryan's caregivers began to offer him various soft foods, such as cereal and pureed fruit. He learned to use his mouth to remove foods from a spoon and to swallow solids. Later, Ryan learned to use his hands to hold his bottle or a piece of toast to chew on. At the same time, his muscles developed so that he could sit up to eat in a high chair.

Ryan began to drink from a cup when he was about eight months old. Soon after, he became interested in feeding himself with a spoon. His first efforts with these new implements were very messy, but he obviously enjoyed the experience. At the same time, he became more skillful at grasping small pieces of food in his fingers.

While Ryan was a toddler, his caregivers gradually introduced a wider variety of foods into his diet. As long as his food was cut into small pieces, he was able to eat independently. By age two, Ryan was sitting in a chair at a child-sized table and chatting with the other children while he ate.

Ryan's improving coordination has enabled him to master more complex tasks during his preschool years. He can now pour drinks from a small pitcher and use a serving spoon to transfer food from a serving bowl onto his plate. He can use a blunt plastic knife to cut cheese or spread peanut butter on bread. He can also spear food with a fork, open many food packages, and carry food and utensils to and from the table. His caregivers give him opportunities to try as many skills as possible, while remaining close by to offer assistance. Observing Ryan's latest skills helps them coordinate his meals with his rapidly progressing development.

1. Like that of other young infants, Ryan's diet at age three months consisted of liquids. How was this suited to Ryan's motor ability at that stage? What other physical characteristics of young infants limit them to fluid nourishment?

_____

_____

_____

2. Which gross motor skills did Ryan use when he sat in his high chair, drank from a cup, and ate with his fingers and a spoon? Which fine motor skills did he use?

_____

_____

_____

_____

3. Give examples of some intellectual and social skills a group of four-year-olds could learn from eating lunch together. What could a caregiver do to encourage the development of these skills?

_____

_____

_____

_____

4. How do Ryan's improving self-feeding skills demonstrate his increasing independence over the period from infancy to age four?

_____

_____

_____

_____

5. Ryan's parents and caregivers recognize the importance of letting him learn to feed himself. Yet they also want him to get all the nutrients he needs. How can they coordinate these two goals?

_____

_____

_____

_____

Introducing Solid Food in an Infant's Diet

Read the passage below and answer the questions that follow.

Tina was changing four-month-old Sam's diaper when his mother arrived at the child care center to pick him up. Tina told Mrs. West that Sam had had a fine day and that there were no problems to report. While she finished dressing him, she continued chatting with his mother.

"I was wondering when you'd like us to begin feeding Sam some solid foods. Have you thought about that yet?" she asked.

"No, not really," replied Mrs. West. "When do you begin with the other children?"

Tina responded, "We don't begin at the same age for every child. We discuss each child's readiness with his parents. Often, the baby's doctor makes suggestions about when to offer solid foods. We follow the parents' plan."

"Do you think Sam is ready yet?" asked Mrs. West.

"Most babies are ready for soft pureed foods, or semisolids, between four and six months of age. Sam's beginning to sit up with support, which he needs to do to eat from a spoon. I see no reason why he shouldn't try solids now." Tina snapped Sam's overalls and handed him to his mother.

Mrs. West looked concerned. "I just switched Sam from breast-feeding to bottle-feeding six weeks ago when he began coming here. Now that he's finally enjoying his bottle, I'd be sorry to take it away and offer him a spoon."

Tina reassured her, "There's no need for Sam to give up the bottle yet. He could continue drinking formula as usual. You could just offer him a few spoonfuls of smooth cereal, once a day, to help him get used to eating that way. Then you could gradually introduce some other pureed foods. Most babies enjoy the new experience. Why don't you ask Sam's pediatrician about it? Even if you don't begin right away, you could come up with a plan. When you do begin, we can coordinate Sam's meals here with the foods you're feeding him at home."

"That sounds fine," said Mrs. West. "But tell me, if all the infants here are following their own schedules for new foods, how do you keep track of what to feed them? It must get awfully busy when several babies are hungry at once."

Tina smiled. "We don't try to remember all those details without help because it does get very busy. In the kitchen area, we keep a chart, which I update every week, with information from the parents. We also keep a record in each child's file. The record keeping takes a little extra time, but it's important to make sure that these early eating experiences are healthful and pleasant for each child."

Application Activity to Use with Chapter 6 ■ ■ ■ **125**

1. Do you think it was wise for Tina to ask Sam's mother now about starting Sam on solid food? Why or why not?

_____

_____

_____

_____

2. Why did Tina suggest cereal as a first solid food for Sam? What type of cereal should Sam try first? What foods should he be offered next?

_____

_____

_____

_____

3. When Sam begins eating solid food, does Tina need to know what he eats for supper at home? Why or why not?

_____

_____

_____

_____

4. Suppose Tina and Mrs. West agree that Sam should start solid foods when he is $4^1/_2$ months old but, when Tina tries feeding him cereal, Sam spits it all out. What should Tina do?

_____

_____

_____

_____

5. Sam can continue drinking from a bottle while he starts eating solid food. When and how should Sam's parents start replacing the bottle with a cup?

_____

_____

_____

Toddlers' Nutrition and Self-Feeding

Read the passage below and answer the questions that follow.

Eighteen-month-old Jenna is enrolled in the toddler class at the Great Beginnings Child Care Center. Like many toddlers, Jenna has become a challenge for her caregivers at mealtime. Jenna insists on feeding herself, adamantly refusing to be fed by a caregiver. She likes to use a spoon, but little of the food actually makes it into her mouth because she has not yet mastered using the spoon as an eating utensil. Jenna enjoys throwing food from her plate onto the floor, and she takes great pleasure in rubbing food into her hair. She is unpredictable about what she will eat on any given day.

Midori, a caregiver at the center, has given up trying to predict Jenna's food preferences. Instead, she has focused on ways to make mealtime less of a battle and more of a nutritional experience for Jenna.

At each meal, Midori begins with very small portions and only puts one food at a time on Jenna's plate. If Jenna eats what is served, Midori serves more of that food before moving on to another food. Midori has noticed that Jenna plays with food mainly when she does not want that food or when she has had enough to eat. Serving small portions of one food at a time has cut down on the amount of food that ends up on the floor or in Jenna's hair.

Midori uses two spoons to serve soft food. She gives one to Jenna to hold while she uses the other to scoop food. She then trades the spoon holding the food for the spoon Jenna is holding. Jenna puts the spoon holding the food in her mouth by herself. Midori and Jenna trade spoons throughout the meal. Jenna enjoys the game and successfully feeding herself. Midori is pleased because with this technique more food actually ends up in Jenna's mouth. She plans to use this approach less often as Jenna's motor skills improve.

Another good strategy that Midori has used is increasing the amount of finger foods she serves. Jenna is quite able to feed herself these foods.

Midori feels she is satisfying Jenna's increasing need for independence and her nutritional needs by using these techniques. Mealtime is still a messy time, but this is to be expected. The amount of mess is more manageable, and there are far fewer battles over who controls the intake of food.

1. How do toddlers' relationships with their caregivers change as they learn to feed themselves?

_____

_____

_____

2. What similarities do you see between toddlers' attempts to feed themselves and their play activities?

_____

_____

_____

_____

3. Give some suggestions for preparing foods for toddlers. How would you prepare both hard and soft foods to suit toddlers' coordination and stage of development? What would you do to make the food attractive to toddlers?

_____

_____

_____

_____

4. Suppose you are about to serve a meal to a two-year-old. The meal consists of bread, cheese cubes, pear slices, yogurt, green beans, and apple juice. How would you prepare the child and the eating area? What utensils would you provide?

_____

_____

_____

_____

Name _____ Date _____ Class _____

Food Preferences

Read the passage below and answer the questions that follow.

Leilani runs an early morning class at the Southwinds Preschool. The children in this group arrive early and eat breakfast together. Then they play until the rest of the children arrive. Leilani glances around the tables and notices that five-year-old Charles is not eating. She kneels beside him and asks, "Charles, may I help you get some breakfast?"

"No, thanks," he replies. "I don't like any of this food."

Leilani suggests, "Let's make sure you know about all the choices. We have two kinds of cereal today—cornflakes and oatmeal—two kinds of juice—apple and orange—milk, bagels, and this big plate of fruit. Would you like to choose something to eat and a drink to go with it?"

Charles responds with a frown, "No, I don't like that kind of cereal. It's too plain. I like sweet cereal and some kinds that have different colors. And I don't like bagels."

Leilani offers to get Charles a piece of fruit and a cup of milk, but he just shakes his head. She knows it will be a long time before the children's midmorning snack and Charles may feel hungry soon if he skips breakfast. "Charles, I have an idea," she says. "Remember the shapes you cut out of clay yesterday? I noticed how well you cut things with a knife. Why don't you take one of these plastic knives and slice half a banana or some strawberries to put on a bowl of cereal? That would make your cereal sweet and colorful. In fact, if you would slice some fruit for me, too, we could eat our cereal together."

Charles looks doubtful, but he reaches for a knife with one hand and some fruit with the other. He keeps busy for some time, slicing bananas and strawberries. He prepares a bowl of fruit and cereal for himself and one for Leilani. Nevertheless, he eats only two bites of fruit and cereal and drinks only half a cup of apple juice. When the breakfast hour ends and Charles heads off for his next activity, Leilani calls after him, "Thanks for the cereal, Charles. It was delicious!"

1. Suppose Charles ate no breakfast at all. How would his nutrition for the day be affected?

_____

_____

_____

_____

2. Charles seems to like sweet foods for breakfast. Do you think Leilani should explain to him why those foods are not good for him?

_____

_____

_____

_____

3. What should Leilani do if Charles occasionally skips breakfast? Should she react differently if he refuses to eat breakfast for two weeks in a row?

_____

_____

_____

_____

4. Suggest some explanations for how children develop a preference for foods high in added sugar. Which causes could be avoided or prevented?

_____

_____

_____

_____

5. How do you think Leilani should deal with Charles the next time the same breakfast items are served?

_____

_____

_____

_____

Vegetarian Diets

There are many types of vegetarian diets and reasons why families choose to adopt them. Some vegetarians eat plant foods and dairy products, whereas others include eggs in their diet. Still others add fish or poultry to the list of foods they eat. The strictest vegetarians (called vegans) eat only foods from plant sources. They eat no meat, dairy foods, or eggs. Regardless of the diet, however, a vegetarian regimen avoids the use of particular foods. Is such a plan a good idea for growing children? Two views on this issue are presented below. Read the passage and answer the questions that follow.

VIEW I. Some people feel that it is unwise for young children to follow a vegetarian diet because it eliminates certain foods. They believe that serving children the widest possible variety of foods is the best way to ensure that children receive all the necessary nutrients in the proper amounts.

An important component of any meal, particularly for children, is the protein content. Meat, eggs, and dairy foods contain all nine of the essential amino acids and, therefore, complete proteins. Preparing meals that contain complete proteins without foods from these categories requires specific combinations of foods that contain incomplete proteins. Omitting entire categories of foods reduces the variety in a person's diet and limits the number of complete protein sources available.

The vitamins and minerals provided by a particular diet are also an important consideration. Meat and eggs are among the best sources of both iron and vitamin B_{12}. Dairy products are the best sources of calcium and vitamin D. Avoiding these food categories can result in deficiencies of these important nutrients. Vegan diets, in particular, do not supply all the nutrients needed by children.

VIEW II. Some people believe that vegetarian diets are quite acceptable for young children, as long as they are well planned nutritionally. Most of the essential nutrients can be found in plant foods, and vitamin and mineral supplements can be used to augment those that are missing or are needed in greater quantities.

The careful planning required to ensure adequate nutrition in vegetarian meals may seem daunting for families unaccustomed to it. However, many familiar dishes that contain no meat are highly nutritious. Following a vegetarian diet on an ongoing basis encourages families to discover many meatless dishes that are healthful and easy to prepare.

Families on vegetarian diets should work with their health care providers to ensure the protection of their children's nutritional status and general health. This is particularly important for families that follow vegan diets. With adequate guidance and attention to nutritional values, many vegetarian diets can be adapted to suit families with young children.

1. Some vegetarian diets include dairy products, whereas others do not. How would the growth and development of children be affected if they follow a diet that excludes dairy products?

_____

_____

_____

2. If parents registering their child for child care mention that they are vegetarians, what questions should the caregiver ask?

_____

_____

_____

3. Plan a lunch menu for a vegan child. Include a source of iron and a source of calcium.

_____

_____

_____

4. What advice would you give to parents who are vegans and are deciding whether to raise their child on a vegan diet? What factors should they consider in their decision?

_____

_____

_____

Name _____ Date _____ Class _____

Identifying Hearing Problems

Read the passage below and answer the questions that follow.

Three-year-old Charlene Jefferson has been coming to the Midtown Child Care Center for several weeks. This is her first experience in a child care situation. Leroy, her teacher, has noticed that Charlene does not seem to be adapting well, and he is concerned.

Charlene appears to have the most difficulty with group activities. She seems restless; for example, she never sits still when Leroy reads a story to the class. She rarely participates in conversations with the other children, and when she does, she often alarms the others by shouting at them. However, she does occasionally play side by side with one or two other children.

From time to time Charlene's lack of cooperation becomes a problem, and Leroy takes her aside to discuss it. Charlene is always much calmer during these sessions and seems to welcome the personal attention. She listens patiently, then she smiles and nods when Leroy asks whether she feels ready to join the class again.

Leroy keeps notes about Charlene's behavior and mentions his concern to the center's director, Polly. Polly spends a morning observing Charlene in class and agrees with Leroy that Charlene's behavior is worrisome. They decide to meet with Charlene's parents to share their concern.

Charlene's parents are surprised to learn that Charlene is not participating in class activities and that she seems so restless. They explain that she is generally easygoing at home and enjoys many of the same activities that she is impatient with at school. They offer to take her to her pediatrician for a checkup, just in case the problem has a medical cause.

A week later Charlene's father reports to Polly that the doctor discovered a problem with Charlene's hearing. She has difficulty hearing individual voices when there is a great deal of background noise. Charlene will be taught some hearing techniques and may be fitted with a hearing device. The doctor has also written down some suggestions for ways that the teachers can help Charlene participate in the class, such as seating her close to the teacher during storytelling. Leroy and Mr. Jefferson agree that knowing about Charlene's condition will enable them both to help Charlene enjoy school.

1. How would an undiagnosed hearing problem interfere with a child's participation in school activities?

_____

_____

_____

2. Why do you think a hearing problem might become apparent in a school situation when it has gone unnoticed at home?

_____

_____

_____

_____

3. What information should the teacher have about Charlene's hearing problem?

_____

_____

_____

_____

4. What do you think a teacher could do to accommodate a child with a minor hearing problem in class?

_____

_____

_____

_____

5. Should Leroy discuss Charlene's hearing problem with the rest of the class? Why or why not?

_____

_____

_____

_____

Name _____ Date _____ Class _____

Caring for Mildly Ill Children

Child care providers are sometimes asked to accept mildly ill children for child care. Should this be allowed? The paragraphs below discuss this question from different points of view. Read the passage and answer the questions that follow.

VIEW I. Mildly ill children generally should not attend child care. An illness that produces only minor symptoms may be highly contagious. Minor symptoms may turn out to be part of the early, contagious stage of a more serious illness. Some illnesses remain contagious even during the recovery stage. The same illness that produces only minor symptoms in one child could cause more serious symptoms in another person. Even if mildly ill children are isolated from other children, their caregivers are exposed to the illness.

A child who is mildly ill often needs rest to recover fully. The child may also be in a weakened condition and susceptible to other diseases. For these reasons, the child would benefit more from remaining at home than from participating in the regular activities of a child care program.

VIEW II. Mildly ill children can be included in the child care setting under certain conditions. A child should only attend if he or she feels well enough to do so and there is no risk of infection to others. Some illnesses, such as middle ear infections, are not contagious. A child whose illness is past the contagious stage does not pose a serious hazard to others. Chicken pox, for example, is no longer contagious about six days after the rash appears. Some illnesses also cease to be contagious in response to medication. Conjunctivitis and strep throat are no longer communicable 24 hours after treatment begins. However, it is important that medication be continued as prescribed, and parents would need to make arrangements with caregivers to see that this is done.

Accepting mildly ill children in child care would allow working parents to reserve their own absences from work (or alternative child care arrangements) for occasions when their child is seriously ill. A child who is only mildly ill might feel most comfortable amid the familiar surroundings of the child care center as she completes her recovery. Caregivers could monitor the child closely and communicate with her parents if symptoms worsen.

1. What role would a center's health consultant play in defining a policy about accepting or excluding mildly ill children from the program?

_____

_____

_____

2. Suppose a child care center agrees to accept mildly ill children for care. What information should parents provide when they bring a mildly ill child to the center?

_____

_____

_____

_____

3. The second viewpoint mentions accommodating the needs of families. Do you think that the first viewpoint also considers factors that are important to families? If so, what are the factors?

_____

_____

_____

_____

4. Do you think policies regarding accepting or excluding mildly ill children from child care should specify different criteria for infants and toddlers than for preschoolers and school-age children? Why or why not?

_____

_____

_____

_____

Name _____ Date _____ Class _____

Playground Safety

Read the passage below and answer the questions that follow.

Pam was out on the playground with her preschool class when she heard a loud cry behind her. She spun around and saw Peter crumpled on the ground beneath the climber. As she ran toward him, his crying continued in waves.

After calming Peter down, Pam determined that he had a scraped elbow. She told the other teachers that she was taking him to the office to use the first-aid supplies. In the office, she told Linda, the school director, about Peter's fall. Linda headed out to the playground to assist with Pam's group.

After school, Pam stopped in the office to tell Linda that she was concerned about the climbing equipment. "Peter is the second child in my class to fall from that climber in two weeks," she explained.

Linda asked her, "What do you think is causing the problem? Is it the equipment or the way the children are using it?"

Pam replied, "Both, I think. The top of the frame is a little too high, and only half of the children can handle it well. Also, the children tend to crowd together up there. They seem to like it, but it is quite challenging."

Linda considered the problem. "Climbing is a good skill for preschoolers to work on," she noted. "If your group enjoys that piece of equipment, maybe there is something we can do to make it safer. Could you limit the number of children allowed up there at one time?"

"I think so," Pam answered. "The whole group was worried about Peter after he fell. I could explain that we want to prevent more accidents."

Linda continued, "I could also ask the parent playground committee whether they could provide some extra sand or wood chips under that climber. An additional layer would decrease the height from the top and provide extra cushioning for any falls."

"That sounds like a good idea," said Pam.

"Why don't we plan to discuss this at the next staff meeting?" said Linda. "We can find out how the other classes are doing on that climber. Meanwhile, let me know how these ideas work with your class."

"Fine," Pam answered. "I think I'll explain the new rule to the children tomorrow, while Peter's accident is fresh in their minds."

1. How would you explain and enforce a rule allowing only three preschoolers at a time on a piece of equipment?

_____

_____

_____

2. What other steps could Linda and Pam have taken to prevent any further falls from the climber?

_____

_____

_____

_____

3. Suppose that later in the year Linda considers letting the toddler group use the preschoolers' playground occasionally. What precautions should she take regarding this piece of equipment?

_____

_____

_____

_____

4. Give an example, other than crowding, of how preschoolers might use playground equipment improperly.

_____

_____

_____

_____

5. Give an example of an equipment problem, other than height, that could be a safety hazard for preschoolers.

_____

_____

_____

_____

Field Trip Safety

Field trips enrich children's school experiences. However, taking children away from the child care center on a field trip means leaving the center's childproof environment. The paragraphs below discuss the safety implications of field trips for young children from different points of view. Read the passage and answer the questions that follow.

VIEW I. Field trips present potential hazards for groups of children and may not be appropriate for very young children. An indoor setting may include such hazards as unprotected stairways and accessible electrical appliances. An outdoor setting may have broken or unstable playground equipment, sharp sticks, animals, poisonous plants, or open access to a busy road.

Transportation to and from field trips also raises safety concerns. Walking trips expose children to pedestrian hazards, including accidents at crossings. Motor vehicle trips run the risk of roadway accidents.

It may be difficult for teachers to supervise children in an unfamiliar setting. Children are easily distracted when surrounded by new sights and sounds. Teachers should only plan field trips with children who are mature enough to observe safety instructions.

VIEW II. Field trips can be organized to protect the safety of children while enriching and reinforcing the curriculum. The key to a successful field trip is careful planning. The route and destination for a trip should be inspected, and the location should be free of any serious hazards. If extra adult supervision is needed, parents or additional staff members should be present on the trip. All adults should be familiar with safety precautions, such as the use of car seats, and any special requirements, such as preventing children from petting animals.

Children can also be prepared in advance. Class discussions about safety and the planned activity can help children follow instructions and increase the benefit they gain from the trip. The activities planned during a trip can also protect children's safety. If there are too many hazards to allow children to explore a site freely, organized group activities with adequate supervision can be designed and carried out.

1. Suppose a preschool class was planning a walking trip to a local nature center, but the route was found to have too many hazardous intersections. What other options could the teachers consider?

_____

_____

_____

2. How could teachers prepare children for a field trip to help protect the children's safety during the trip?

_____

_____

_____

_____

3. Do you think field trip destinations need to meet all the safety criteria enforced in classrooms? Explain your answer.

_____

_____

_____

_____

4. How does the age range of the children in a group affect the safety precautions necessary for a field trip?

_____

_____

_____

_____

5. Give an example of how a field trip could enrich a preschool curriculum.

_____

_____

_____

_____

Lesson Planning

Read the passage below and answer the questions that follow.

Amanda sat in the children's library flipping through a book on health and hygiene. She was planning to discuss dental health with her preschool class, and she was looking for ideas. She found it easy to identify the concept she wanted to present: It is important to take good care of our teeth. As she thought about how to illustrate the concept, however, she realized that it included several distinct topics. She decided the best approach would be a series of separate lessons. Each lesson could focus on a different topic. She was eager to keep the discussions within the children's attention span and to offer plenty of variety in the related activities.

Amanda knew that most of the children followed some dental care routine at home. Therefore, she could expect them to be familiar with the subject although they might not be very knowledgeable. She also felt that there was a limit to the amount of information they could absorb at this stage. For example, she was certain the children would be able to understand that sugar harms teeth, but she knew they would not understand the chemical reactions involved. Bearing this in mind, she selected topics for her lessons. She came up with three: (1) Nutrition—How foods affect our teeth, (2) Personal Hygiene—Keeping teeth clean to prevent decay, and (3) Professional Dental Care—How the dentist cares for our teeth.

Amanda also drew up a list of activities to illustrate the topics. This list included calcium-rich/low-sugar snacks (such as grilled cheese on toast and yogurt with fruit) for the children to prepare, a verse about toothbrushing to add to a song they already knew, an activity in which the children would make wide-mouthed puppets and cardboard toothbrushes, a puppet show with the new puppets, and a visit from a dentist. She drafted a note to send home with the children, outlining the topics she planned to discuss so that the children's families could follow up. She also made a list of necessary supplies and things she would need to do to prepare for each activity.

Before leaving the library, Amanda checked out a stack of storybooks relating to teeth. She began to feel that this piece of the curriculum was falling into place.

1. What aspects of Amanda's lessons provide repetition and predictability for the children?

_____

_____

_____

2. What instructional objectives could Amanda set for her three topics?

_____

_____

_____

_____

3. How would Amanda's dental health lessons help children develop a positive self-concept?

_____

_____

_____

_____

4. What other subject areas overlap with Amanda's topics and activities?

_____

_____

_____

_____

5. Do you think dental health is an appropriate concept for a preschool class to discuss? Why or why not?

_____

_____

_____

_____

Communicating with Parents

Read the passage below and answer the questions that follow.

Francine was planning to hold conferences with the parents of the children in her preschool class. In preparation, she posted a conference schedule outside the classroom. She sent a note home with the children, asking parents to sign up for a specified time and offering to make special arrangements for any parents who could not come at any of those times.

Francine also sent home a note inviting parents to come to school with their child on a day of their own choosing. She explained that parents could use the day in any way they would like, such as sharing a special activity with the class, helping to celebrate their child's birthday, or just observing or participating in a normal school day. Parents unable to come during the day were welcome to choose a date to send in something from home, such as a favorite family food or souvenirs from a family trip.

A week before conferences were to begin, the conference schedule was nearly full. One parent, Mr. Raymond, sent a note saying that he could not make any of the conference times but that he was free during his lunch hour. Francine arranged for another teacher to stay with her class during lunch so that she could meet with him. Mrs. Preston said that she was unable to get a babysitter for her two children during the conference. Since parents of children in other classes had the same problem, the center set up a babysitting room where two staff members would supervise children who needed care during conferences. Francine called Mrs. Preston to tell her and posted a note to inform the other parents.

Meanwhile, replies to the parent participation requests began coming in. Most parents chose to come on their child's birthday, but some chose other days, such as holidays they would be celebrating. Many parents had suggestions for activities that they would like to share with the children, such as cooking events or craft projects. Francine was encouraged by the response. Between her discussions with parents about scheduling conferences and their offers to participate in class activities, she felt that she was already getting to know the children's parents—and the conferences hadn't even begun.

1. Francine sent information to parents in notes that went home with the children. Do you think this is an effective way of communicating with parents? Why or why not?

_____

_____

_____

2. How did Francine take into account the demands on parents' time, such as work commitments, in her communications about conferences and parent participation in class?

_____

_____

_____

3. How did Francine indicate to Mr. Raymond and Mrs. Preston her willingness to help overcome their difficulties in attending conferences?

_____

_____

_____

4. What should Francine do if one child's parents fail to sign up for a conference?

_____

_____

_____

5. How do you think Francine should prepare for the conferences?

_____

_____

_____

Answers

Chapter 1

Study Questions

1. d   2. h   3. b   4. f   5. c   6. i
7. a   8. g   9. e

10. Nutrition, health, and safety. They cannot be isolated from one another, and any change in one affects the others.

11. Proteins, carbohydrates, fats, vitamins, minerals, and water.

12. A person needs different amounts of nutrients at different stages in life.

13. It determines whether children will reach their full potential over time.

14. Socioeconomic—people with low incomes may not be able to afford a variety of foods; cultural—different ethnic groups emphasize certain foods and food preparation styles; emotional—emotions may cause people to overeat or lose interest in eating; education—people with sound nutrition information are likely to make wise food choices.

15. They can provide meals that supply a variety of foods and nutrients, or they can monitor what children bring to eat.

16. The foods a person eats, heredity, and environment.

17. Eye color, blood type, and skin color.

18. Physical, economic, social, and cultural settings.

19. An environment that is clean, comfortable, and stimulating.

20. They can take action to prevent the spread of disease, learn to recognize the signs and symptoms of various childhood diseases, know what to do when a child is sick, and exchange important health information with parents.

21. The safety of the children in their care.

22. Knowing the most likely sources of danger.

23. Mechanical suffocation, aspiration and choking, burns, electrical shock, poisoning, falls, drowning, motor vehicle injuries.

24. Act safely themselves, set and enforce rules that help children behave safely, and teach children about safe behaviors.

25. Practicing what to do in an emergency, knowing whom to contact and how to communicate with them effectively, and knowing basic first-aid procedures.

26. Each one has an effect on the others. Heredity and the environment have effects on nutrition, health, and safety. Some inherited disorders affect the body's ability to maintain good nutrition or health; environmental conditions may make certain settings unsafe.

Application Activity

1. Picking up toys is a precaution against falling; walking with food in one's mouth poses a risk of aspiration and choking.

2. Eliza could establish regular handwashing times (such as before meals) for the whole class. She could praise children who wash their hands at other appropriate times (such as after using the bathroom), remind those who forget to do this, and let the children see her washing her own hands.

3. Insisting that children finish all their food could encourage overeating, which might develop into a lifelong habit. However, encouraging them to try each item helps them learn to eat a wide variety of foods with different nutritional benefits.

4. Children who share their food will miss out on some of the sources of nutrition in their own lunches. They may not replace these sources with something similar from a friend's lunch. Children who eat food prepared for another child may be exposed to foods to which they are allergic. They may eat something they are supposed to avoid for religious or cultural reasons.

5. Eliza encouraged the children to share their thoughts on these issues, she kept her discussions brief, and she saved some topics to cover later. For this age group, she could have used other means of explaining the same points, such as pictures, games, songs, or stories.

Chapter 2

Study Questions

1. g   2. b   3. d   4. a   5. f   6. e
7. c

8. A positive food environment promotes good eating habits and a child's overall enjoyment of food.

9. Make sure that they are suited to a child's body size and level of physical dexterity.

10. Make proper handwashing before and after handling food and eating it a routine; locate food-handling and eating areas far away from toilet and diaper-changing areas; store used tissues, wipes, and diapers in closed containers away from food and discard them daily.

11. Hunger is a physical sensation that signals that it is time to eat; appetite is a desire to eat stimulated by the body's senses.

12. Every two to three hours.

13. This supports the establishment of healthful diets and healthful lifelong eating patterns.

14. Serve cooked foods warm rather than hot; offer a variety of textures; avoid the excessive use of sugars, salt, and fats; offer food in small servings of bite-sized pieces; offer a combination of finger foods and foods to eat with utensils; avoid offering hard, small pieces of food to children under the age of four.

15. If a child repeatedly refuses a food, a caregiver can try substituting a food with a similar nutrient content.

16. They can allow children to make food choices, serve themselves, and clean up after themselves.

17. Talk about each food's qualities before tasting it; offer new foods when children are not tired, excited, or already full; offer one new food at a time.

18. Family resources, family structure, ethnic identity, religious beliefs, education, knowledge of nutrition and health, geographic residence, and emotional factors.

19. Each child's food patterns are learned from his or her family's food culture.

20. Both parents may work; fathers and older siblings may purchase and prepare food and feed children; busy schedules promote a reliance on fast foods.

21. Help children resolve their emotions and find ways to ensure adequate nutrition in the meantime.

22. Respect everyone's food culture, respect similarities and differences in food and the way people eat, try new foods, learn about food from your family, learn about food from your friends.

23. Integrate ethnic and regional foods into their regular menus. Organize food tastings or cooking events with various ethnic or regional foods. Provide utensils for dramatic play involving cooking and eating and read books to children about ethnic foods.

Application Activity

1. Being hungry can interfere with the children's ability to participate in school activities. These patterns could also indicate that the children are not getting enough nutrition, which could be harmful to their health and development. Moreover, the eating habits formed during childhood are often retained into adulthood.

2. Jarrod eats frequent small snacks and no full meals at home. At school he is expected to eat less frequently and to divide his diet into full meals and light snacks; he misses his frequent snacks and feels hungry. Olivia is accustomed to eating breakfast at a time of day when there is no meal scheduled at school. She finds it difficult to eat at an earlier time or wait until the scheduled snack time.

3. Donna's advice for Jarrod is good because he is at a stage of development when he should not need to eat more frequently than every two to three hours. Frequent nibbling of snack foods may not provide all the nutrients that are more likely to be included in full meals, unless great care is taken to plan nutritious items for snacks.

4. It would be helpful to know what Olivia's father offers her for breakfast; perhaps it is a food that she does not like, or perhaps the quantity is overwhelming for her early in the morning. Donna could also ask about the family's evening meal. Do they eat a large meal together? Do they eat late in the evening? These factors could affect Olivia's appetite in the morning.

5. Children who seem tired or complain of headaches or stomach pains might also be hungry. Individual children can be affected by hunger in different ways.

Chapter 3

Study Questions

1. j **2.** k **3.** h **4.** a **5.** e **6.** c **7.** i **8.** f **9.** l **10.** g **11.** d **12.** b

13. They promote growth and development, provide energy, and allow people to maintain health, resist infection, and perform the daily functions of life.

14. No, only three—carbohydrates, fats, and proteins.

15. Sugars are the simplest, smallest form of carbohydrates. Complex carbohydrates break down more slowly and provide a steady supply of sugars. Fiber is a type of complex carbohydrate that aids in digestion.

16. Grains and grain products, nuts, seeds, vegetables, fruits, dry beans, honey, milk, table sugar, other sugars.

17. They carry fat-soluble vitamins, provide essential fatty acids, and improve the appeal of many foods.

18. Cholesterol is part of all body cell membranes and is important to the nervous system. It is needed for the production of bile, many hormones, and vitamin D.

19. At high levels, LDL cholesterol is associated with deposits of cholesterol on artery walls; HDL cholesterol is associated with a lower risk of cholesterol deposits.

20. The body cannot make some fatty acids. Children's bodies need these essential fatty acids to grow normally, and adults' bodies need them to keep skin and other tissues healthy.

21. Because the body needs these amino acids to grow and function normally, but it cannot make them.

22. Meat, poultry, fish, eggs, most dairy foods, legumes, nuts, seeds, grains.

23. Seeds found in the pods of certain plants and used for food; beans, peas, lentils, peanuts, and soybeans.

24. The water-soluble vitamins are the B vitamins and vitamin C. The fat-soluble vitamins are vitamins A, D, E, and K.

25. Vitamin A helps maintain vision at night, maintains healthy skin and mucous membranes, helps white blood cells fight infection, and aids in the development of bones and teeth. Vitamin D works with certain minerals to form and maintain bones and teeth and to help muscles contract and relax.

26. Food provides all the nutrients the body needs for health; supplements do not. Vitamins in food are often better absorbed by the body than those in supplements.

27. Unlike many vitamins, minerals are not destroyed by heat.

28. Calcium works with phosphorus to help build and maintain bones and teeth, aids in muscle contraction, helps transmit nerve impulses, and is necessary for blood clotting. Phosphorus works with calcium to help build and maintain bones and teeth, is necessary for growth and maintenance of tissues, and is used in energy production and the movement of fats.

29. Water helps carry nutrients to the cells, removes the by-products of metabolism, and helps cool the body through perspiration.

Application Activity

1. Foods provide vitamins and minerals and many other nutrients, such as proteins, fats, carbohydrates (including fiber), and water. Foods provide energy.

2. Caregivers should have complete medical information about children in their care, and this could include dietary and nutritional information. However, caregivers should encourage children to eat healthful meals regardless of whether or not the children take vitamin and mineral supplements.

3. Milk contains vitamins B₂, B₁₂, and K and is fortified with vitamins A and D. Dark-green leafy vegetables supply vitamins B₂ and K. Meat and eggs contain vitamin B₁₂. Vitamin A is found in liver and carrots, and vitamin D is found in liver and eggs.

4. Calcium and iron are both important to children's well-being. A child who eats no dairy products might need supplementary calcium. A child with anemia might benefit from iron supplements.

5. The caregiver should explain the risks and benefits of vitamin and mineral supplements and the overall importance of a healthful diet. If the parents have a special concern about the child's health, the caregiver could recommend that they discuss their concerns with their health care provider.

Chapter 4

Study Questions

1. e   **2.** j   **3.** c   **4.** h   **5.** d   **6.** i
7. a   **8.** g   **9.** f   **10.** b

11. Overall fitness, or an optimum physical, mental, and psychological condition.

12. The Recommended Dietary Allowances provide calorie recommendations and suggest the amounts of many key nutrients an average healthy person needs each day.

13. Eat a variety of foods; maintain healthy weight; choose a diet low in fat, saturated fat, and cholesterol; eat plenty of vegetables, fruits, and grain products; use sugars in moderation; use salt and sodium in moderation; if you drink alcoholic beverages, do so in moderation.

14. Six to eleven servings daily. Breakfast cereal, muffins, bread, rice, spaghetti or macaroni, pita bread, rolls, pretzels, or other grain products.

15. Nutrient-dense foods supply plenty of nutrients for their calories; calorie-dense foods supply few nutrients but plenty of calories.

16. Eat fats, oils, and sweets sparingly.

17. Children's small stomachs empty more quickly than adults', and children are less likely to be able to compensate for the discomfort of midmorning hunger.

18. Snacks help provide the calories and nutrients children need daily. Because children have small stomachs, they often cannot satisfy their needs at meals alone.

19. Many pediatricians advise against giving infants whole milk until they are over one year old because of its high protein content and its potential to trigger allergic reactions.

20. They can offer plenty of iron-rich legumes and fortified grain products; include milk, cheese, yogurt, and eggs in their diets; and make sure that they consume enough complete protein.

21. Serving size; servings per container; calories; calories from fat; amounts of total fat, saturated fat, cholesterol, sodium, total carbohydrates, fiber, sugars, and protein; and amounts of vitamins A and C, calcium, and iron.

22. Use liquid vegetable oils when fat is needed; use low-fat cooking methods; skim off visible fat from liquids; drain fat after cooking meat.

23. Remove saltshakers from the table; prepare pasta, rice, cereal, and vegetables without adding salt to the cooking water; limit the consumption of processed meats and high-sodium prepared foods.

24. Sucrose (table sugar), brown sugar, raw sugar, dextrose (glucose), fructose, maltose, lactose, honey, syrup, corn sweetener, high-fructose corn syrup, molasses, or fruit juice concentrate.

25. Nutrients, warmth, moisture, and sufficient time.

26. Washing hands before and after handling food; wearing clean clothes while handling food; tying long hair back; using tongs, scoops, serving spoons, and disposable gloves; cleaning utensils between uses; storing foods away from chemicals and cleaning supplies; storing dry foods in sealed containers off the floor in a cool, dark area; refrigerating perishable foods; cooking meat, poultry, fish, and eggs to the proper temperatures; keeping hot foods hot and cold foods cold until they are served; refrigerating and promptly using leftovers; checking dates on packaged foods.

Application Activity

1. The Food Guide Pyramid is a good resource because it identifies the food groups and shows the relative number of servings needed from each group.

2. The school should offer milk because it provides nutrients, particularly calcium and protein, that are essential for children.

3. Varying the children's lunches provides them with a wider range of nutrients. It gives children the chance to try more foods and develop good eating habits.

4. Parents should know what foods are fed to their children. Some children have food allergies; others come from families that, for religious or other reasons, avoid certain foods. Caregivers need to be aware of these facts and communicate with parents.

5. The teachers should encourage the child to try some of the foods. If she will not eat any of them, the teachers could offer a substitute food (such as some bread or crackers) so that the child will not be hungry. They should also inform the child's parents and, in this case, the director or kitchen staff, who wish to keep track of such reactions.

Chapter 5

Study Questions

1. h **2.** c **3.** a **4.** f **5.** i **6.** d
7. j **8.** b **9.** g **10.** e

11. A developing baby is called an embryo from the second to the eighth week after conception. From the start of the ninth week until birth, it is called a fetus.

12. Cephalocaudal development progresses from head to foot, whereas proximodistal development moves from the center of the body toward the extremities.

13. Tissue differentiation occurs, the fetus's major organ systems begin to develop, the brain begins to form, and the heart begins beating.

14. By the middle of the second trimester.

15. Many organs mature, the eyes open, the lungs complete their development, and the brain develops rapidly.

16. Steady increases in height and weight, steady changes in body shape and proportion, the maturation of organ systems, and the development of motor skills and language skills.

17. Genetic makeup, environment, nutrition, gender, birth order, and state of health.

18. By six months, control head movement and sit up. By one year, pull themselves along with their arms and crawl on their hands and knees. By 1½ years, toddle and walk. During the second year, walk up stairs and kick a ball.

19. Between nine months and one year of age, babies understand the word *no*, often respond to their names, and begin babbling nonsense syllables. A one-year-old may use a few words meaningfully. During the second year, most children become able to name a dozen things, make animal sounds, follow simple directions, and use two-word phrases. Preschoolers start speaking in complete sentences and can listen to and understand simple stories. By age five, children can describe their wants, needs, and daily routines.

20. Diet can help children grow and develop to their own genetic potential. An inadequate diet can limit physical development.

21. Any three of the following: memory, comprehension, reasoning, problem solving, and attention.

22. The development of attitudes, emotions, personality, identity, and social skills.

23. They are needed in reactions that release energy from digested foods to fuel growth. They play a part in the manufacture of amino acids used in building new tissues. Folic acid is needed to make red blood cells and genetic material for all new cells.

24. Calcium and phosphorous provide the strength in bones and teeth; sodium, chloride, and potassium help maintain the water balance of the body.

25. To determine whether a child is getting an adequate and balanced amount of nutrients.

26. Any three of the following: the 24-hour recall method, a food diary, an interview, or a questionnaire.

Application Activity

1. Young infants are not yet able to chew and swallow solids, but they can suck and swallow liquids. At this stage, infants require a fluid diet because their digestive systems are not yet able to break down solid foods and because they need large amounts of water.

2. Sitting up is a gross motor skill that uses many of the large muscle groups in a child's body. Eating and drinking used gross motor movements of Ryan's arm. He also used fine motor skills such as the pincer grasp and other subtle movements of his fingers and hands to hold his cup and spoon and to pick up bits of food.

3. Eating lunch together could help four-year-olds learn the names and characteristics of various foods and improve their ability to share and cooperate. The caregiver could discuss simple nutrition concepts and could model and discuss appropriate table behavior.

4. As a young infant, Ryan was largely dependent on adults. Learning to hold his bottle meant he could drink without assistance. Grasping pieces of food allowed him to eat solids on his own. Learning to use utensils enabled him to scoop, cut, and spear foods and even to prepare some foods for himself.

5. They can provide a varied selection of nutritious foods, present foods in an appealing way, create a pleasant eating environment, and set an example of healthful eating patterns while allowing the child to feed himself.

Chapter 6

Study Questions

1. i **2.** f **3.** g **4.** e **5.** a **6.** j
7. b **8.** h **9.** d **10.** c

11. Weight gain and increases in length and head circumference.

12. Newborns have a suckling reflex that soon gives way to sucking movements. Around the fourth month, infants develop an up-and-down munching movement of the jaws. In the seventh to ninth months, babies can drink from a cup, and at the end of the first year they develop chewing abilities.

13. Between the fourth and eighth months.

14. Exploring new foods is a form of learning and self-feeding helps develop a sense of independence.

15. They smile in response to a smiling face; they recognize their primary caregiver and respond with smiles; they begin to perform deliberate acts to change their environment; they imitate the activities of others; they understand some words and respond to their names; they drop objects to watch them fall; and they begin to feed themselves with a spoon.

16. Specific times during development when children should have appropriate experiences if they are to continue to develop normally.

17. An infant's caloric requirements gradually decrease during the second six months, from about 49 calories per pound of body weight to about 44 calories per pound. This change occurs because an infant's growth slows during this time and more calories are used in activity and fewer in growth and development.

18. Babies should be fed in a quiet, relaxed environment in which caregivers give them their full attention. Ideally, caregivers should cuddle babies during feeding and make eye contact with them.

19. These vegetables contain large amounts of nitrates, chemical substances that babies' immature digestive systems cannot properly digest. Feeding infants these vegetables could result in nitrate poisoning.

20. Because an infant's immature digestive system passes more unchanged proteins into the bloodstream.

21. Advantages: human milk is easily digested by infants, rarely produces allergic reactions, and contains antibodies and other factors that help protect the baby from infections; it cannot be incorrectly prepared or become contaminated; the closeness and physical contact during nursing encourage a strong emotional attachment between mother and child. Disadvantages: breast-feeding mothers must be very cautious about drug and alcohol intake; some viruses can be passed to infants in breast milk; being the sole or main source of nourishment for a baby may be a source of stress for the mother; some women may experience physical discomfort while nursing.

22. The inner core of the bottle gets hot while the outside remains cool. Caregivers might feel the outside of the bottle and believe that the milk is an acceptable temperature when it is actually too hot.

23. One at a time, at intervals of about a week.

24. It rarely causes an allergic reaction, is easily digested, and provides iron.

25. Infants and children should determine how much food to eat; caregivers should be sensitive to children's signals that they have had enough. Insistence that children "clean their plates" may lead to poor eating habits and obesity later in life.

26. Make sure the pieces of food are of a size and shape that will not be aspirated; gradually increase the texture of foods offered to babies; do not leave babies alone while they are eating; let babies touch, smell, and play with their food to learn about it; wash babies' hands before and after they eat; provide child-sized utensils and small food portions.

Application Activity

1. This is a good time to ask because it is the beginning of the average range of ages during which infants become ready to eat semisolid foods. Caregivers should know what parents are planning and can offer suggestions to parents as needed.

2. Rice cereal is usually the first food; it is easy to digest and rarely causes allergic reactions. Individual fruit and vegetable purees are generally offered next.

3. Knowing what foods are eaten at home helps caregivers ensure that only one new food is introduced each week. It may also help determine the cause of any allergic reactions.

4. Tina should tell Sam's parents and wait a week or two before trying solids again. Sam may need more time to develop the mouth patterns needed for swallowing solids.

5. Most infants begin using a cup when they are between six and eight months of age. The cup should be introduced gradually, as bottle- or breast-feedings decrease. It is also important to introduce the cup when Sam is still interested in drinking but not excessively hungry or thirsty. It is best to begin with small amounts of liquid in the cup. These measures will minimize frustration for Sam and his caregivers.

Chapter 7

Study Questions

1. e   2. a   3. c   4. b   5. d

6. Legs grow more rapidly than trunk, and chest grows more rapidly than abdominal areas. This gives the toddler a taller, thinner appearance. Legs remain bowed and short relative to the trunk, but as posture improves and abdominal muscles grow stronger, the toddler begins to look more like a young child.

7. By 18 months, most toddlers can use a spoon and drink from a cup. At two years, spoon-feeding has improved, and most toddlers can handle a glass. By 2½, most toddlers have acquired good rotary chewing skills.

8. Between 12 and 15 months, toddlers use jargoning, a kind of speech gibberish that sounds like sentences.

By 18 months, most toddlers can say 10 or more words. By the age of two, toddlers have a vocabulary of about 300 words. They speak in sentences about 40 percent of the time, and the rest of the time in two- to three-word phrases.

9. Because it shows that toddlers see themselves as individuals with their own needs.

10. They can stop asking questions for which *no* is an answer and phrase questions so that toddlers can choose between two acceptable alternatives.

11. Dark-green leafy vegetables, cooked dry beans, tortillas or tofu processed with calcium, and calcium-fortified fruit juices.

12. Complex carbohydrates; pasta, cereals, breads, rice, beans, and certain vegetables.

13. Because children are at their hungriest in the morning and are most likely to eat well if given appropriate choices and adequate time to eat.

14. Most meals should contain foods from all five food groups. Snacks should contain foods from two or more food groups.

15. Make healthful snacks available throughout the morning or afternoon, allowing the child to help herself when she is ready to eat.

16. Toddlers should be fed five to six times a day at intervals of at least 2 to 2½ hours. Caregivers should allow at least 30 minutes for each meal.

17. It encourages toddlers to experiment with new foods as they watch their caregivers and playmates eat, and it promotes independence because toddlers can begin to help with food service.

18. Toddlers who finish their meals feel a sense of accomplishment. Small portions allow them to assert their independence by asking for more.

19. They can send home information about the food groups and easy-to-prepare lunch menus.

20. Caregivers can cut food into bite-sized pieces; avoid serving foods that are difficult to chew and can block a child's airway; and remind toddlers to eat slowly, chew carefully, refrain from talking while eating, and remain seated during meals.

21. Adults should put other nutritious foods the toddlers like on their plates, even if they don't eat them. Adults should not make an issue of the behavior.

Application Activity

1. Toddlers sit on their own and eat with less assistance than they did as infants. They become more aware of their individual identities and more independent of the caregivers.

2. Manipulating food and playthings exercises the developing fine motor skills. Toddlers learn from exploring the textures, shapes, and other properties of their food and their playthings in much the same way. Most toddler exploration is done orally.

3. Hard foods should be cut into bite-sized pieces; soft foods should be easy to scoop with a spoon. Interesting textures, shapes, and color combinations make food appealing. Foods should also be served warm or cool rather than hot or cold.

4. The child's hands should be washed, clothes protected with a bib, and paper or plastic spread on the floor. The child should be placed in a sturdy child-sized seat or high chair, depending on the child's level of development. A cup and spoon should be provided.

Chapter 8
Study Questions

1. e **2.** c **3.** d **4.** b **5.** a

6. Discuss their findings with the child's parents.

7. A preschooler's head grows more slowly than a toddler's, but the face grows more rapidly and the jaw widens. Legs become longer in proportion to total body length. The spine straightens out and the abdomen protrudes less prominently.

8. Carrying serving dishes to the table; setting the table; preparing certain foods, such as cereal with milk; and cleaning the table.

9. In a calm, nonjudgmental manner to help the children develop a positive self-concept.

10. Recognizing similarities and differences between objects and the ability to follow simple directions.

11. 1,400 calories.

12. 30 percent. Margarine, vegetable oils, meat, fish, poultry, nuts, and dairy products.

13. Iron. Children who drink large amounts of milk may have no appetite left for foods that are rich in iron.

14. Green pepper, broccoli, and brussels sprouts.

15. Meat and meat alternates that are high in salt and fat, such as hot dogs and luncheon meats.

16. Carbohydrates, B vitamins, and iron.

17. Vary the texture, shape, and color.

18. Serve it with familiar foods, talk about the food with the child, enjoy the food yourself, present a neutral response to the child's acceptance or refusal of the food, and continue to offer it to the child.

19. It gives the children some control over what they eat and helps them develop a sense of independence and autonomy.

20. Do not add sugar or sweeteners to vegetables, fruits, or cereal; do not serve candy, sweetened beverages, or refined baked goods; for birthdays, suggest that parents bring more nutritious snacks than cakes or cookies.

21. The key principles of variety, balance, and moderation apply over time and not necessarily to each and every meal and snack.

22. They can talk with children about television commercials and explain some of the misinformation given there.

23. They can involve the children in planning and preparing what they will eat.

Application Activity

1. To get enough nutrients and calories, he would have to eat more than usual at his other meals and snacks. He would probably be quite hungry and do this without any special encouragement.

2. It would be better not to comment on Charles's food preferences. She could explain the effects of sugar on health in a general sense at another time.

3. Skipping meals occasionally is not harmful; but skipping breakfast regularly could indicate a problem. Leilani should speak with Charles's parents if this happens. They might be able to explain his lack of interest in breakfast (early morning snacking on cookies, for example) or might want to consult his health care provider about possible causes.

4. Eating habits of family and friends, restaurant meals, and media advertising could expose children to such foods. Children might develop the preference after repeatedly tasting the food. Parents and caregivers can avoid this by not serving foods high in added sugar.

5. She should encourage him to try them again; each attempt may help him to learn to enjoy the foods. However, she should continue to avoid negative comments about his preferences.

Chapter 9

Study Questions

1. b   **2.** h   **3.** g   **4.** c   **5.** a   **6.** e
7. j   **8.** d   **9.** i   **10.** f

11. Inadequate diet, illness or physical condition that prevents the body from using certain nutrients, certain medications, physical disabilities.

12. Because children must both replace red blood cells that are destroyed through normal processes and make additional red blood cells to increase the volume of blood their bodies need as they grow.

13. Combining foods high in vitamin C with iron-rich foods and combining iron-rich vegetables with meat.

14. Lack of sunlight from staying indoors excessively or living in a high-pollution area, having dark skin, being a breast-fed baby of a vitamin D–deficient mother, following a vegan diet, drinking unsupplemented milk.

15. Less than 10 percent of children born to normal weight parents are obese; a high percentage of obese children have at least one obese parent; identical twins raised separately tend to have similar weights; adopted children have body weights closer to those of their biological parents than their adoptive parents.

16. No direct link between the two has been clearly established. However, time spent watching television is time not spent in more vigorous physical activities, and children who watch television tend to snack more.

17. Ensure that activities stress individual abilities instead of competition and provide ample time for active outdoor play.

18. By making sure they maintain a normal weight, reduce salt (sodium) intake, get regular exercise, and avoid stress.

19. Because an infant's immature intestines allow more proteins from food to pass into the bloodstream, where the immune system may react to them; avoid the food that causes it.

20. Cow's milk, eggs, wheat, corn, soy, peanuts, chocolate, citrus fruits, strawberries, fish, shellfish.

21. Work with the child's parents to find an appropriate diet, alert other parents who may be sending in snacks for the children, request ingredient lists from parents for homemade foods, obtain parental permission before serving the child any foods not prepared at the center.

22. Eliminate the problem food from the child's diet.

23. Evaluating a developmentally delayed child's nutritional needs may be difficult; some developmentally delayed babies may have difficulty sucking, chewing, or swallowing; the age at which a developmentally delayed child is ready to accept new foods will probably differ from the average age for other children; children who eat laboriously because of a developmental delay may need more time for each meal.

24. Because they are growing more rapidly than full-term babies and have smaller stores of nutrients in their bodies.

25. Breast-feeding has value not only for nutritional reasons but also because of the close physical contact between mother and child and the immune protection supplied by breast milk.

Application Activity

1. The vitamins and minerals in milk, particularly vitamin D and calcium, are essential for proper growth. Children who do not eat dairy products run the risk of deficiencies and poor development if they do not get these nutrients from other sources.

2. The caregiver should ask what foods are excluded from the child's diet and how any missing nutrients are to be supplied. If the diet is very limited, the caregiver might also ask whether the parents have discussed it with a health care professional. Caregivers should, however, be aware that people from cultures that are traditionally vegetarian are not likely to need guidance about vegetarian diets and children's health.

3. Calcium is found in broccoli; spinach contains both calcium and iron. Legumes and enriched breads contain iron. One possible menu: a peanut butter sandwich on enriched bread, broccoli spears or a spinach salad, and fruit juice.

4. Parents should consider the types and amounts of nutrients necessary for children's growth and the limited sources of some of these in a vegan diet. If they decide to raise their child on a vegan diet, they should consult a health care professional about ensuring that the diet provides adequate amounts of as many nutrients as possible and using vitamin and/or mineral supplements to provide the remainder.

Chapter 10

Study Questions

1. c 2. h 3. e 4. b 5. d 6. f
7. j 8. g 9. a 10. i

11. They are used to monitor normal development and to identify health problems for diagnosis and treatment.

12. Health history, immunization record, medical examination results, list of emergency contacts, records of height and weight, screening results or other medical information, daily observations of caregivers.

13. It authorizes staff members to make decisions about a child's medical treatment in an emergency if a parent or guardian cannot be reached.

14. Helps ensure the health of each child and the group, makes children more aware of the importance of their own health, can assure parents that their children are receiving careful attention from the staff.

15. The caregiver should work closely with the center director, following center policies in caring for the sick child and obtaining medical assistance if necessary.

16. Basic first aid and cardiopulmonary resuscitation.

17. A child may make great efforts during visual tasks, such as leaning forward, squinting, rubbing the eyes, or holding an object very close or very far away to see it, or he or she may complain of frequent headaches.

18. The name for several eye disorders caused by improper muscle control of the eyes; the eyes do not work together properly, producing double vision or crossed or drifting eyes. Strabismus patients may need to wear eyeglasses or an eye patch, and they may need to do eye exercises.

19. Language development may be delayed, and the ability to learn may be adversely affected.

20. Asthma, seizure disorder, heart defects, hemophilia, sickle cell disease, diabetes, cystic fibrosis, PKU, fetal alcohol syndrome.

21. The child suddenly finds it difficult to breathe. Breathing out takes a great effort and may be accompanied by wheezing. Breathing in also becomes difficult, and the child may be in considerable pain.

22. Because their blood does not clot properly, severe or even fatal blood loss could occur.

23. It requires all facilities open to the public to provide accommodations for people who have disabilities.

24. Immunization information, a childhood disease history, and often the results of a medical examination.

25. Bend the knees, hold the child or object close to the body, and lift with the leg muscles rather than with the back and shoulders.

Application Activity

1. A hearing problem would create difficulty with any activity that involves speech or sound, such as storytelling, discussions, or group projects.

2. At home, there may be less background noise and parents might speak individually to the child. In the noisier school environment, the child's limited hearing would become more apparent.

3. The teacher needs to know the limits of the child's hearing, whether she needs special assistance during the day, and whether there are any restrictions on her activities.

4. The teacher should follow recommendations from parents or health care providers; this could include working individually with the child or seating her close to the speaker during presentations.

5. Yes, he should explain to the other children how they can help Charlene understand their speech. He could also discuss the special arrangements the teachers will make to help Charlene during activities such as storytelling and explain any hearing techniques or devices Charlene may use.

Chapter 11

Study Questions

1. d 2. h 3. c 4. b 5. j 6. a
7. g 8. e 9. f 10. i

11. They are more likely to be exposed to various diseases because they come into contact with more people; level of development increases risk (immature immune systems, mouthing everything, no control of bowels or bladders); parents may send children to child care when they are not entirely well; caregivers may come to work when they are not well.

12. Viruses are the smallest variety of pathogens, or disease-causing organisms. They invade healthy cells and use the cells' resources to reproduce themselves.

13. Immunization exposes a person to a weakened or killed strain of a virus. The body forms antibodies against the virus without getting the disease.

14. The nature of the disease, whether the person has other medical conditions, whether the person eats well and gets enough rest.

15. By respiratory droplets, by fecal-oral contamination, by direct contact, by body fluids.

16. Frequent handwashing and washing and disinfecting toys.

17. It is a bacterial disease that causes flulike symptoms. It is dangerous because it can lead to serious infections or inflammations of the throat, joints, lungs, blood, and coverings of the brain.

18. They can practice proper diaper changing and disposal, disinfect surfaces that could be contaminated with feces, and keep food preparation and serving areas separate from diaper-changing areas. If possible, caregivers who change diapers should not prepare food.

19. Giardia is an intestinal parasite that can cause several symptoms, including diarrhea, gas, weight loss, and fatigue. Most giardia infections originate with contaminated water sources, and the disease is spread through fecal-oral contamination.

20. The eyes become red and itchy and discharge fluid. It can be treated with antibiotics; the person affected is no longer contagious 24 hours after treatment begins.

21. They can eliminate hats from dress-up play, launder dress-up clothes often, discourage children from sharing hairbrushes or touching each other's heads, provide individual cubbies for storing coats and other clothes, and educate parents about the parasites.

22. HIV is spread by the introduction of infected body fluids directly into the body of an uninfected person. This usually occurs during sexual activity, but it may also take place through a break in the skin. The virus can also be transmitted from an infected pregnant woman to her unborn child. Hugging, shaking hands, or sharing a bathroom with an infected person will not transmit HIV because the virus cannot live outside the body.

23. Polio, diphtheria, pertussis, hepatitis B, mumps, measles, rubella, tetanus, and Hib disease.

24. Arrange cots and cribs so children sleep head to foot, provide adequate space and ventilation, keep room temperatures between 65° and 75° F (18.4° and 23.9° C) in the winter and 68° and 82° F (20° and 27.8° C) in the summer, clean air conditioners and vaporizers regularly, air out rooms daily, provide an individual storage cubby for each child's personal belongings, separate diapering areas from eating and food preparation areas, locate the diapering area near running water, remove dirty diapers and trash daily, provide a space where children who become ill can be kept apart from other children.

25. When sick children will be sent home, when and how the center will notify parents if children become sick during the day, the policy for readmission after an illness, the circumstances in which medication will be administered, the circumstances under which emergency care will be sought, how parents will be notified about exposure to communicable diseases, how parents should notify the center about reasons for absence.

Application Activity

1. The health consultant could advise the school's director about symptoms, periods of communicability, and recovery stages for particular diseases; indicate the importance of specific symptoms for children of various ages; and suggest criteria and safeguards for administering medication.

2. The parents should tell the center about their child's symptoms, whether the child has seen a doctor, the doctor's diagnosis, details about any medicines prescribed, and where they can be reached if needed.

3. Yes, the concern about the risk of contagion and the recommendation of rest and isolation for ill children would be important to families.

4. Infants have less mature immune systems, and diseases spread quickly among children who are not toilet trained and who mouth toys. Some symptoms are also more serious for infants and toddlers; for example, diarrhea poses a greater risk of dehydration for very young children. An illness policy might include some distinctions based on these differences, but it is simpler to have one policy that applies to all children.

Chapter 12

Study Questions

1. c   2. g   3. a   4. e   5. h   6. b
7. d   8. f

9. The development and widespread use of antibiotics, vaccines, and other medical advances.

10. Motor vehicle accidents; failure to use child restraints or to use restraints properly.

11. Infants cannot direct their movements to get away from anything that interferes with their breathing.

12. They cannot stop excess liquid from flowing out of a bottle, and without help they may choke and breathe the liquid into their lungs.

13. Between the ages of one and four; children's abilities are not adequate to deal with their environments or they move quickly and get into situations where adult supervision is inadequate.

14. When the center is short of staff, when caregivers are tired or under stress, in the late morning and late afternoon when children are hungry and tired, on field trips, and when the center's routine is disrupted.

15. Rearward if the child weighs less than 20 pounds; forward if the child weighs 20 pounds or more.

16. In the five- to nine-year-old age group. Children of this age spend more time outdoors, and many fail to observe traffic safety rules.

17. To prevent unintentional injuries in infants and toddlers, a caregiver must limit their access to hazards. With preschoolers, supervision and physical barriers can be combined with safety education to prevent injuries.

18. Because it may be a way to be accepted by their peer groups.

19. Failure to follow traffic laws and failure to use proper equipment, particularly bicycle helmets.

20. Smoke alarms, carbon monoxide alarms, fire extinguishers, emergency lighting, window guards,

handrails and nonslip treads on stairs, safety gates, safety plugs for electrical outlets, safety glass.

21. Toys should be safe, durable, developmentally appropriate, and washable. Cloth toys should be made of flame-retardant fabric. Toys should not have sharp or broken edges or small pieces that can be swallowed.

22. Fruit-scented markers, commercial dyes that contain chemical additives, epoxy and other solvent-based glues, aerosol sprays.

23. Equipment present should be age-appropriate; playgrounds should be fenced; all areas of the play space should be visible; large play structures, especially swings, should be surrounded by adequate space; the surface of the playground beneath and around equipment should be covered with an adequate depth of an impact-absorbent material.

24. Pea gravel, sand, and wood chips are less expensive but require more upkeep and renewal than rubber matting.

Application Activity

1. Explain the reason for the rule, propose a method for choosing groups of three, and set a time limit for each group if necessary.

2. They could create rules about the type of play allowed (such as "No hanging" or "No climbing to the top"), instruct teachers to stand near the equipment to supervise safe play, or place the equipment off limits if it is too hazardous.

3. She should consider whether the toddlers are capable of using the equipment safely; if not, they should not be allowed to use it. Extra supervision might be needed to keep toddlers away from the climber.

4. Climbing up the ramp of a slide, standing on a swing, and throwing sand are examples of improper use of playground equipment.

5. Broken or weakened equipment of any kind would be a problem, as would sharp edges, unstable supports, crooked swings, slides that are too steep, or large gaps between climbing rungs.

Chapter 13

Study Questions

1. e   2. a   3. b   4. i   5. c   6. j
7. f   8. d   9. h   10. g

11. Establish a physically safe environment, consistently enforce age-appropriate safety rules, provide alert supervision, educate children about safety issues.

12. Young children lack the ability to generalize and apply one rule to several different situations.

13. They should precede the activity with a discussion of how to use the equipment safely; ensure that extra adults, such as parent volunteers, are present; limit the number of children using the equipment at any given time; take time to explain the activity and classroom rules to parent volunteers.

14. Protect the other children in the class, perhaps by isolating the aggressive child; if behavior appears to signal other problems, the teacher should consult the director about referring the child and family to professional help.

15. Children should take turns on equipment, the number of children on a piece of equipment at one time should be limited, and no shoving or "pretend fighting" should be allowed.

16. Children have a greater skin surface area relative to their body weight, and water is lost through the skin.

17. It is a rope that has knots tied in it every few feet and is used to provide safety on walking field trips. An adult holds each end of the rope, and each child is assigned a knot and instructed to keep her or his hand on it at all times while walking with the group.

18. Arranging the building so that anyone entering must pass a receptionist, requiring parent visitors to sign in and wear a visitor's badge, locking all outside doors except one (locked doors must readily open from inside), and requiring parents to sign a form indicating who may remove their children from the center.

19. Not to talk to strangers, not to go with strangers, and to scream for help if a stranger attempts to pick them up.

20. Parents, health care professionals, and alternative emergency contacts if parents are not available in an emergency.

21. The name and age of the injured person; a description of the injury and the circumstances under which it occurred, including where and when; the names of the supervising adult and other witnesses; the action taken in response to the injury.

22. Immerse the hand in cold water. If the skin is broken, cover the hand with a clean cloth and seek medical help.

23. Try to stop the bleeding with continuous pressure with a clean cloth on the wound. Keep the child warm and watch for signs of shock. If the bleeding does not stop or is severe, call for medical help.

24. Neglected children usually show more physical signs of their condition than do abused children. They may be hungry, dirty, tired, inappropriately dressed, or constantly ill.

25. The name, address, and age of the child; the extent of the child's injuries; the names and addresses of the parents; the identity of the offending adult, if known; often, your name and address.

26. The difference between good touching and touching that makes them uncomfortable; the idea that their bodies are their own and they can decide who touches them and where; the difference between good secrets and secrets that make children uncomfortable or involve threats.

Application Activity

1. Investigate other destinations in the neighborhood, organize a parent car pool, invite the director of the nature center to come and talk to the class, run a class project based on a nature center display.

2. Describe the location to children, explain the events planned, assign each child a particular adult to travel with, have a procedure for what children are to do if they get separated from the group.

3. No. Children spend more time, and generally have more freedom, in class than they do on a trip, so more safety criteria must be met. The site for the trip should be safe enough that children do not encounter any hazards during the course of their visit.

4. Very young children need to be supervised more closely, more adults are needed, and appropriate child seats must be used for automobile travel. Older preschoolers and school-age children can follow safety instructions more effectively.

5. Field trips can provide experiences not found in the school environment, such as seeing how foods are grown, watching professionals at work, or visiting sites of cultural, historic, or scientific interest.

Chapter 14

Study Questions

1. f   2. a   3. d   4. e   5. c   6. b

7. To promote healthy behavior during the preschool years and to motivate children to develop good nutrition, health, and safety habits for the rest of their lives.

8. Building a positive self-concept, skills acquisition, knowledge acquisition, and attitude development.

9. They can give the child many opportunities to master skills and to feel successful.

10. Physical, emotional, social, intellectual, and creative skills.

11. Unbiased, inclusive attitudes toward others and an openness to new experiences.

12. They can treat all children with respect and affection regardless of their skin color, gender, or ethnic background.

13. Offer variety, plan developmentally appropriate material, keep ideas simple, use repetition and predictability, strive for inclusiveness.

14. Answers will vary but should include a selection of activities from which children can choose. A lesson about fruits, for example, might offer children the choice of painting a picture of a fruit, tasting different kinds of fruit, or categorizing fruits by color.

15. They can provide opportunities for children to experience information again and again in new and progressively more challenging ways. Each lesson plan should review and then build on concepts that have already been introduced.

16. Teachers should try to understand the reasons for the withdrawal and make efforts to include these children without forcing participation. Some children may want to practice a skill with an adult before trying it with their peers.

17. Choose an overall idea or concept, choose a topic to illustrate the concept, prepare instructional objectives for the activity, select activities that achieve the objectives, and evaluate the lesson plan.

18. Answers will vary: foods have different names, flavors, and textures; foods come from plants and animals; people need a variety of foods to stay healthy; exercise is fun and good for you; many sicknesses are caused by germs passed from one person to another; children should be cautious around strangers; sharp objects must be handled safely.

19. Topics should clearly explain or demonstrate the concept for the age group; they should fit the developmental level as well as the needs and interests of the group; appropriate materials and equipment should be available; the whole class should be able to get involved; there should be multicultural aspects.

20. It should describe the specific content to be covered or the specific behavior that is expected, and it should be measurable or observable.

21. To determine whether the instructional objectives were met, whether the lesson met the needs of the learners, whether the planned activities were appropriate and helpful, whether the teacher was effective.

22. At the end of each day because the day's events will be fresh in the teacher's mind; also on a monthly or quarterly basis to see how the curriculum may be revised to accommodate new situations.

23. Maintaining balance in the program, making connections to other subject areas, considering timing factors, staying flexible.

Application Activity

1. The healthful snacks repeat the theme of foods that are good for teeth; toothbrushing is featured in the new verse of the familiar song, the puppet making, the puppet show, and the dentist's presentation.

2. (1) Children will identify one food that is good for teeth and one that is harmful; children will name one nutrient (sugar) that is harmful to teeth. (2) Children will demonstrate effective toothbrushing technique. (3) Children will name two steps that occur during a visit to the dentist.

3. Learning how to take care of themselves gives children a sense of pride and accomplishment.

4. Nutrition, cooking, health, hygiene, music, crafts, dramatic play, and learning about professionals in the community.

5. Yes, because it is a subject that all children can participate in and it is important to develop good dental care habits early.

Chapter 15

Study Questions

1. b 2. a 3. e 4. d 5. c

6. The family's cultural background, the family's level of education, the amount of money available for food, and the personal preferences of family members.

7. Registration forms, pre-enrollment questionnaires, conferences with parents, orientation programs.

8. Information—both positive and negative—about the child who is being cared for and about the family.

9. Answers will vary but should include a teacher response that restates the parent's feelings or concerns, such as the following:

   Parent: "Tom doesn't seem to be eating much lunch lately."

   Teacher: "You're concerned that he's not getting enough to eat during the day."

10. These are good times for exchanges of information between the caregiver and the parents.

11. By writing a note or a letter, calling parents, or scheduling a parent-teacher conference.

12. To avoid questions or misunderstandings about what was communicated.

13. Length of naps, number of times diapers were changed, kind and amount of food eaten, activities, difficulties or accomplishments noted during the day.

14. Positive information, such as the child's general adjustment to the program and daily experiences, progress in various areas, new accomplishments and positive changes, and examples of how the curriculum can meet the child's developmental needs.

15. A handbook, fliers, newsletters, a bulletin board, a resource center.

16. Information about the school's activities, projects, and upcoming events as well as public health and safety information.

17. Parents can place the menu on the refrigerator or memo board so they can discuss with their children what is being served each day.

18. An open house for explaining the school's curriculum, a parenting workshop, a presentation by a nutritionist, a workshop or a seminar, a potluck dinner.

19. Seeing children in their home settings can provide caregivers with many insights about children and their families. Children enjoy home visits from caregivers.

20. They enable parents to get to know one another and to share information with one another as well as with the school.

21. Caregivers can show parents that they like and appreciate their children and that they are concerned with their children's welfare.

22. Through observation, presentations, or activities; volunteering in the classroom or on their own time at home; donating materials; and being part of a cooperative.

23. Such recognition gives parent volunteers a feeling of satisfaction and invites the participation of other parents in activities.

Application Activity

1. Notes to parents provide a useful written record of the information; they should be delivered directly to parents if possible.

2. She offered to make special arrangements for conferences to suit parents, and she offered a way for parents who were not able to come in during the day to contribute to class activities.

3. She made a special effort to solve each parent's difficulty, and she communicated personally with them.

4. She could speak to them to make sure they are aware of the conferences, describe the purpose of the conferences in a positive tone, and ask whether they have a problem with attending.

5. She could prepare to describe the program and daily routine, review each child's progress, and note any questions she would like to raise with parents about their children.